Novel Developments in Gastroenterology

John Libbey Eurotext
127, avenue de la République
92120 Montrouge
Tél. : 33 (0) 1 46 73 06 60
e-mail : contact@john-libbey-eurotext.fr
http://www.john-libbey-eurotext.fr

John Libbey Eurotext Limited
42-46, High Street
Esher
Surrey
KT10 9QY
United Kingdom

© John Libbey Eurotext, 2006
ISBN : 2-7420-0651-6

Il est interdit de reproduire intégralement ou partiellement le présent ouvrage sans autorisation de l'éditeur ou du Centre Français d'Exploitation du Droit de Copie, 20, rue des Grands Augustins, 75006 Paris.

Novel Developments in Gastroenterology

Edited by
P. Malfertheiner
L. Lundell
G. Tytgat

Combined EAGE, ASNEMGE, EDS, IDS, EAES
Postgraduate Course 2006
Berlin, October 21-22

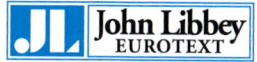

Contents

Foreword
G.N.J. Tytgat, P. Malfertheiner, L. Lundell VII

I – Mucosal Damage and Repair

Basic mechanisms of drug-induced mucosal damage and repair
C. J. Hawkey 3

Drug-induced oesophageal mucosal injury
C. Cellier 5

Spectrum of drug-induced gastric damage
A. Lanas 9

Drug-induced small/large bowel injury
C. Beglinger 15

Prevention of mucosal injury: whom, when, and how?
J. Regula 21

Role of endoscopy in diagnosis and therapy of drug-induced UGI bleeding
J. Sung 25

Role of medical therapy in drug-induced bleeding
J. Mössner 29

Is the COX-1, COX-2 hypothesis obsolete?
R.H. Hunt 35

II – Novel Developments in Gastroenterology. Medical and Surgical Viewpoints

1. Non acid and duodeno-gastro-oesophageal reflux

Non acid and duodenogastroesophageal reflux. Proofs of concepts and definitions
D. Sifrim 45

The role of bile and pepsin in the pathophysiology and treatment of gastroesophageal reflux disease
J. Tack 53

Impedance pH monitoring
R. Tutuian... 63

Non-acid and duodeno-gastro-oesophageal reflux: therapeutic options
J. P. Galmiche.. 67

2. What is really new in the diagnosis and management of intestinal neuropathies and motility disorders

Irritable bowel syndrome
G. Boeckxstaens... 73

Systematic review of sacral nerve stimulation for faecal incontinence and constipation
M. A. Kamm et al... 75

3. Techniques and indications for minimally invasive procedures

Conventional *versus* robot-assisted thoraco(laparo)scopic esophagolymphadenectomy for esophageal cancer
J. Boone, I.H.M.B. Rinkes, R. van Hillegersberg.. 77

4. New diagnostic tools: ready for clinical application?

Evaluating new diagnostic technology: a case of the Law of the Hammer?
P.M.M. Bossuyt.. 81

Positron emission tomography *versus* computed tomography in gastrointestinal malignancies
M. Westerterp, J.J.B. van Lanschot... 83

Magnetic resonance cholangiopancreatography *versus* endoscopic retrograde cholangiopancreatography in HPB diseases
M. Delhaye... 89

Addendum

Chronic intestinal pseudo-obstruction syndrome
O. Goulet

Foreword

A highlight of the EAGE postgraduate program is obviously the postgraduate course at the time of the annual UEGW meeting. Whenever possible and appropriate, the EAGE looks for strategic alliances in the organisation of this event.

Two main topics of high current interest have been chosen for the 2006 Berlin postgraduate course: Mucosal damage and repair and Novel developments in gastroenterology. Medical and surgical viewpoints.

Drug-induced mucosal damage is of immense importance in gastroenterology. It is imperative that clinicians understand how these lesions come about, what the sometimes devastating consequences are and what can be done to prevent or to treat such calamities. Drug-induced damage is bound to increase in the future as the population ages and polypharmacy becomes the rule instead of the exception. Hopes for improvement were shattered when the longterm consequences of COX-2 inhibition became available. Is the COX-1/COX-2 concept truly obsolete?

Several issues will be discussed by European experts is the second part on Novel developments. What the clinician should know about non acid, weakly acid or biliary reflux will be discussed in depth. Novel developments of gastrointestinal neuropathies and motor disorders will concentrate on IBS, pseudo-obstruction and fecal incontinence. Our surgical colleagues will certainly be interested in novel minimally invasive procedures. Finally all will learn from a critical analysis of novel diagnostic imaging modalities.

Remains for me to thank my EAGE program collaborators, the representatives of ASNEMGE, particularly Prof. C. Hawkey, and the representatives from EDS. Together with all of them, I like to thank most sincerely all presenters for their willingness and expertise. Last but not least, flowers for Mrs Jonsson for organisational help.

May the Berlin 2006 postgraduate course be a source of enrichment for all of us, to the ultimate benefit for those we care for.

Prof. Emer. G.N.J. Tytgat
also on behalf of EAGE representatives
Prof. P. Malfertheiner and **Prof. L. Lundell**

I

Mucosal Damage and Repair

Basic mechanisms of drug-induced mucosal damage and repair

C. J. Hawkey

University of Nottingham, UK

Gastrointestinal mucosal injury can arise as a result of the toxicity of physicochemical trauma (*e.g.* alcohol), interference with mucosal defence mechanisms (*e.g. via* inhibition of prostaglandin synthesis by NSAIDs) and by alterations in immune reactivity (often abrogation of immune tolerance) (*e.g.* TNBS colitis). Direct mucosal defence mechanisms operating to a greater or lesser extent throughout the gut involve mucosal blood flow and dependent processes of ion and mucus secretion. In the stomach and duodenum, sodium bicarbonate is secreted and plays an important role in neutralizing acid diffusing through the mucus layer. These processes have been shown to be highly dependent on synthesis of prostaglandins but, because of the importance of mucosal blood flow, can also be maintained by other vaso dilators. Of particular importance are nitric oxide and CGRP dependant enteric neuronal responses. Mucosal defences can also be abrogated in ways that do not involve inhibition of prostaglandin synthesis or altered blood flow. An example is the barrier breaking properties of salicylates which lead to enhanced acid back diffusion that can be shown to occur in humans using tonometry.

Localisation of NSAID associated injury varies according to individual drugs. In animal studies, non aspirin NSAIDs result in predominantly distal intestinal injury whereas the effect of aspirin is in the stomach. This probably relates to high drug concentrations in the terminal ileum as a result of recirculation of some non aspirin NSAIDs. Although aspirin also undergoes enteopathic recirculation, it is in the form of metabolites. Type C gastritis, although not apparently the cause of clinical symptoms, gives an intriguing insight into the effects of NSAIDs. Most chronic users who are not infected with *Helicobacter pylori* have type C gastritis. The only other significant cause is a duodenal gastric bile reflux. Whether the presence of re-circulated NSAIDs within bile is responsible is not known.

There is some controversy about whether COX-1 inhibition alone is sufficient to cause gastroduodenal injury. Most NSAIDs are combined inhibitors of COX-1 and COX-2. Studies in animals suggest that dual inhibition is required for significant injury. This may be because COX-2 is induced in response to initial COX-1 inhibition to provide a compensatory source of protective prostaglandins. Whether this is important in humans is less clear but an endoscopic study has suggested that rates of ulceration with aspirin and rofecoxib are greater than would be expected from their effects alone.

Barrier function is strongly influenced by the metabolic activity of myofibroblasts which lie subjacent to and in close proximity to epithelial cells. This has been shown for colonocytes and may also occur in the stomach, although a lack of suitable models has precluded direct testing. Myofibroblasts produce basement membrane components and one function of these appears to be to facilitate rapid repair by cellular migration (epithelial restitution) of minor breaches following injury.

Mucosal defences cannot be seen solely in terms local processes. Growing data suggest that the metabolic activity of symbiotic and probiotic bacteria in the colon has far reaching effects mediated by circulating pharmacological agents and by re-circulating immunocytes. In addition, human and animal studies involving sex-mismatched stem cell transplants show that myofibroblasts and other cells involved in mucosal defence appear to be renewed from circulating stem cells. Whether these are haemopoetic or mesencymal stem cells is not entirely clear.

Drug-induced oesophageal mucosal injury

Christophe Cellier

Department of Gastroenterology, European Georges Pompidou European Hospital, Paris, France

A variety of medications have been reported to cause oesophageal injury. More than 1,000 cases of pill-induced oesophageal injury have been described in the litterature, but this number is probably a gross under-representation of the problem. Pill-induced oesophageal injury is also associated with many underlying diseases inducing increased contact time between the medication and the oesophagus.

Risk factors that predispose to pill-induced oesophageal injury

The main factors that predispose to to pill-induced oesophageal injury are:

– decreased salivary flow (aging, sicca symptoms, anticholinergic medications),
– disorderered oesophageal motility (achalasia, strictures, ineffective oesophageal motility, aging),
– disordered local anatomy (dysphagie lysonia, aortic aneuvrysm, enlarged left atrium),
– medications formulations (capsule, sustained-released formulations, large tablets, odd-shaped pills),
– medications affecting the tone of the lower oesophageal sphincter (benzodiazepines, adrenergic agonists, theophylline, opoid analgesics, calcium channel blockers...),
– ingestion of the medication in supine position (bed time).

Diagnosis and clinical features of drug-induced oesophageal injury

Usually patients present with sudden-onset chest pain, dysphagia and odynophagia; most symptoms occur within a few hours to days after taking the medication. The patients will improve once the drug is removed. A prolonged dysphagia caused by development of stictures may be observed for alendronate, ferrous sulfate, NSAIDs or potassium chloride. The more common medications causing pill-oesophagitis are: alendronate, quinidine, tetracycline, doxycicline, potassium chloride, ferrous sulfate, mexiletene.

Upper GI endoscopy typically shows focal areas of erythema, erosion, and ulceration. Drug induced injury is a strong possibility if discrete erosions occurs in areas away from the Z line.

Specific medications causing oesophageal injury

Alendronate

Post-marketing experience has associated oral amino-biphosphonates with upper gastrointestinal intolerance and oesophageal injury including ulceration, stricture, and perforation. Endoscopic studies have identified differences among aminobiphosphonates in their potential for injury, which is thought to arise from prolonged mucosal contact with intact tablet. Administrating the medication with tap water in an upright position can reduce oesophageal stasis and minimize mucosal exposure. Novel protected formulation of alendronate that houses the active drug in an inert shell may be less likely than standard alendronate to induce severe mucosal injury.

NSAID – induced oesophagitis

There are few reports of NSAID – induced oesophagitis. However most NSAIDs groups, including low-dose aspirin, have been reported to injure the oesophagus, especially in patient with GERD.

Antimicrobial medications

Doxycycline and tetracycline are the two most frequently responsible drugs-induced oesophagitis in that class of drugs. The majority of patients present with severe dysphagia, chest pain and odynophagia, and most show superficial ulceration or inflammation in the mid-oesophagus without strictures.

Radiation-induced oesophageal injury

Radiation therapy results in both acute and chronic oesophageal injury. Doses greater than 5000cGy may predispose to stricture formation and chronic radiation injury. A number chemotherapeutic agents may exacerbate the effects of radiation, including cyclophosphamide, 5-fluoroouracil, and cisplatin.

Conclusions

Drug-inducest oesophageal injury is probably underrecognized. Most injury occurs because of an increased contact time between the medication and the oesophagus due to disordered anatomy, poor salivary flow, and impaired motility. In general, prevention of pill-induced injury is the optimal therapy. Simple instructions to patients who are at risk are mandatory. This can be achieve by the patient's drincking of water with any medication, avoidance of lying down for at least 30 minutes after taking the medications.

References

- Arora A, Murray JA. Iatrogenic esophagitis. *Curr Gastroenterol Rep* 2000?; 2: 224-9.
- Lanza F, Hunt R, Thomson R, Provenza M, Blank M. Endoscopic comparison of esophageal and gastroduodenal effects of risedronate and alendronate in postmenopausal women. *Gastroenterology* 2000; 119: 631-8.
- Marshall J, Thabane M, James C. Randomized active and placebo-controlled endoscopy study of a novel protected formulation of oral alendronate. *Dig Dis Sci* 2006; 51: 864-8.
- O Neill J, Remigton TL. Drug-induced esophageal injuries and dysphagia. *Ann Pharmacother* 2003; 37: 1675-84.

Spectrum of drug-induced gastric damage

Angel Lanas

University of Zaragoza, Spain

A large number of drugs have been associated with dyspepsia, but the evidence indicates that non-steroidal anti-inflammatory drugs (NSAIDs) are the only class of drugs that are frequently associated with both symptoms, and a wide range of lesions in the gastro-duodenal tract. NSAIDs are amongst the most commonly used medications worldwide for the treatment of pain and inflammation. Traditional NSAIDs inhibit both isoforms of cyclooxygenase (COX), the enzyme which transforms arachidonic acid into prostaglandins and thromboxanes which are involved in inflammation, pain and platelet aggregation. COX-1 is expressed in most tissues producing prostanoids that are involved in defence and repair of the gastrointestinal (GI) mucosa, in platelet aggregation and thrombosis, and in some central nervous system pathways regulating pain. COX-2 is expressed constitutively in some tissues including vascular endothelium, kidney and the central nervous system but is induced in most tissues and leucocytes in response to inflammatory stimuli.

The main benefit of non-selective NSAIDs derives from their anti-inflammatory and analgesic effects, while the main adverse effects are seen in the GI tract. COX-2 selective inhibitors (coxibs) have a significantly better GI safety profile but recent data have raised concern over long-term use being associated with an increased risk of cardiovascular (CV) thrombotic events. Inhibitors of COX also share other potential benefits (*e.g.* cancer preventive effects) and adverse effects (*e.g.* hypertension). Furthermore, aspirin, an irreversible inhibitor of COX-1 and platelet aggregation, has specific and unique effects within this class. Aspirin at doses lower than 300 mg/day acts as a selective COX-1 inhibitor and has cardio-vascular protective effects although it carries dose dependent risks of GI complications.

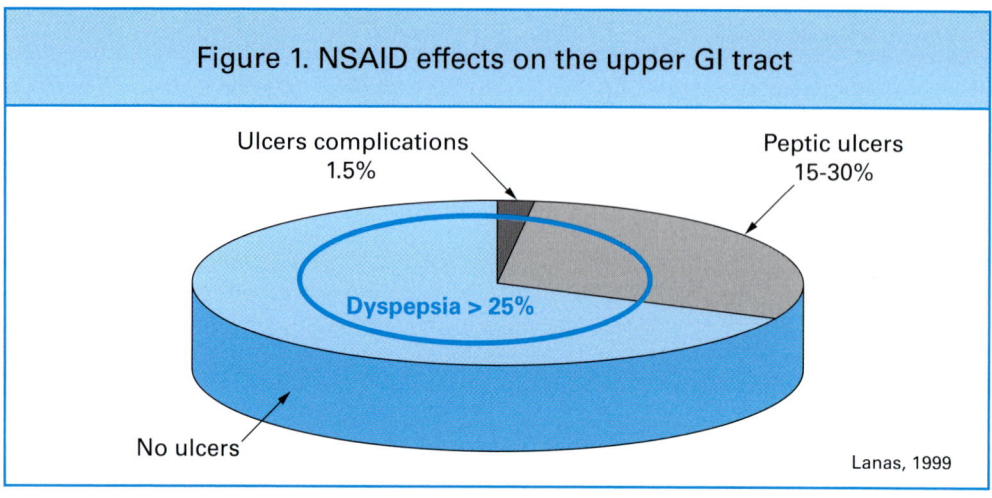

Figure 1. NSAID effects on the upper GI tract

Lanas, 1999

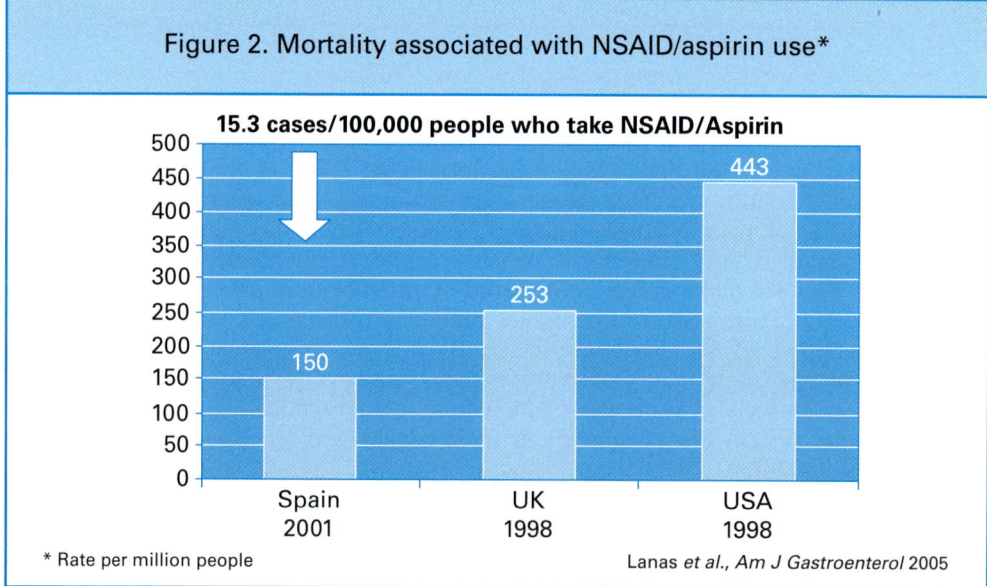

Figure 2. Mortality associated with NSAID/aspirin use*

15.3 cases/100,000 people who take NSAID/Aspirin

* Rate per million people

Lanas et al., Am J Gastroenterol 2005

Non-selective NSAIDs and the gastroduodenal tract

NSAIDs can adversely affect both the upper and/or lower GI tract, although most GI safety studies have focused on upper GI events. Endoscopy studies, often focusing on sub-clinical markers, are abundant, but the clinical relevance is unclear, since endoscopic lesions are common but seldom correlate with symptoms or serious clinical outcomes. These endoscopic lesions include petechia, erosions and ulcers. Thirty to fifty per cent of patients taking NSAIDs develop gastro-duodenal lesions but the majority of these lesions are trivial (petechia and erosions) and asymptomatic in most cases and disappear or reduce in number with continued use.

Serious events including upper GI bleeding, perforation and gastric outlet obstruction occur in approximately 1-1.5% of patients within the first 12 months of treatment with a non-selective NSAID. When symptomatic ulcers are included this figure rises to 4-5% of patients treated over one year. ASA is also associated with both gastric and duodenal ulcers and upper GI complications occur even with the lowest dose of 75 mg/day. The worst GI outcome results in death, but mortality data associated with NSAIDs treatment are scarce. A recent large nation-wide study in Spain reported 15.3 deaths/100,000 NSAID/aspirin users. Other studies have reported that one in 1,200 patients taking NSAIDs for at least 2 months dies from gastroduodenal complications. In the US, another widely quoted report from the early 1990s estimated deaths at 16,500 cases per year.

Upper GI symptoms occur in up to 50% of patients taking non-selective-NSAIDs, and some 5-15% of patients with rheumatoid arthritis discontinue NSAIDs because of dyspepsia.

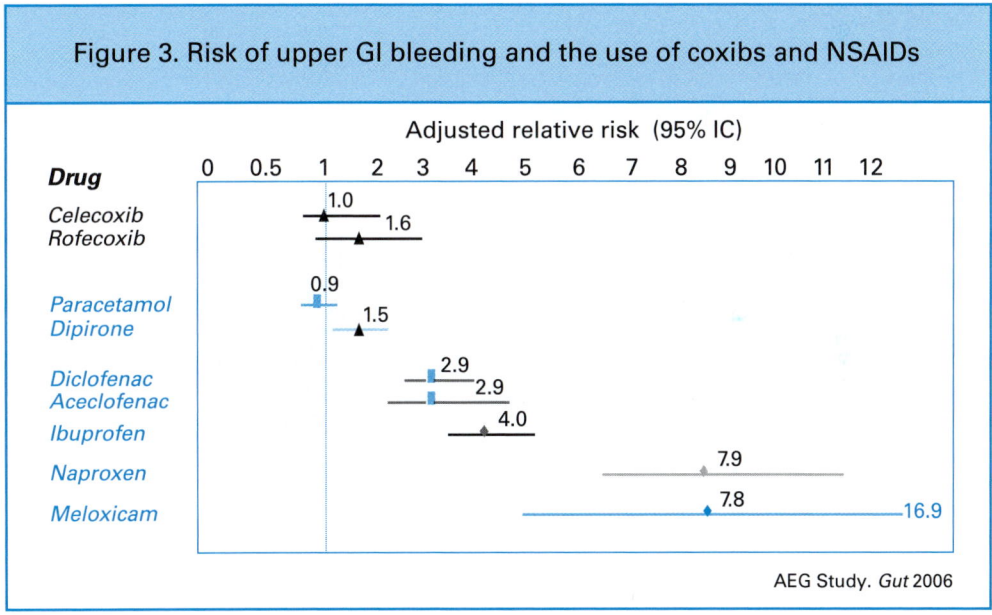

Figure 3. Risk of upper GI bleeding and the use of coxibs and NSAIDs

AEG Study. *Gut* 2006

COX-2 selective inhibitors and the gastroduodenal tract

Coxibs have an improved upper GI safety profile, extensively shown in endoscopy and clinical outcomes studies. Two big outcomes trials show that high-dose rofecoxib and high-dose lumiracoxib were associated with a 50-70% reduction in upper GI complications when compared to ns-NSAIDs. Although the incidence of adverse events with coxibs increased in relation to the presence of risk factors, the differences from non-slective NSAIDs was maintained in subgroups of patients with and without risk factors for ulcer complications. The CLASS study did not confirm the benefits of high-dose (800 mg/day) celecoxib *vs* NSAIDs, probably because of the concomitant use of low-dose aspirin by

22% of patients. However, a recent meta-analysis confirms that celecoxib at any dose was associated with significantly less clinical ulcers and bleeds than ns-NSAIDs. Moreover, the results of another large outcomes study with celecoxib, the SUCCESS I study confirmed the significantly better safety profile of celecoxib (200-400 mg/day) compared with diclofenac and naproxen in 13,274 patients with osteoarthritis. Upper GI complications were seen significantly less in the celecoxib treated patients (0.1/100 patient years) compared with the ns-NSAIDs (0.8/100 patient years). Second generation coxibs, such as etoricoxib, have greater selectivity for COX-2 and also show improved GI tolerability compared with ns-NSAIDs in patients suffering from rheumatoid arthritis or osteoarthritis. Recent epidemiological studies have confirmed that coxib use is associated with a small or no increased risk of upper GI bleeding.

Concomitant ASA and NSAID or coxib treatment carries measurable risk of an adverse upper GI event. In addition to the CLASS study, evidence from the TARGET and SUCCESS I trial, endoscopy and epidemiological studies indicate that low-dose aspirin increases further the risk of upper GI bleeding in NSAID users and attenuates the GI benefits of coxibs.

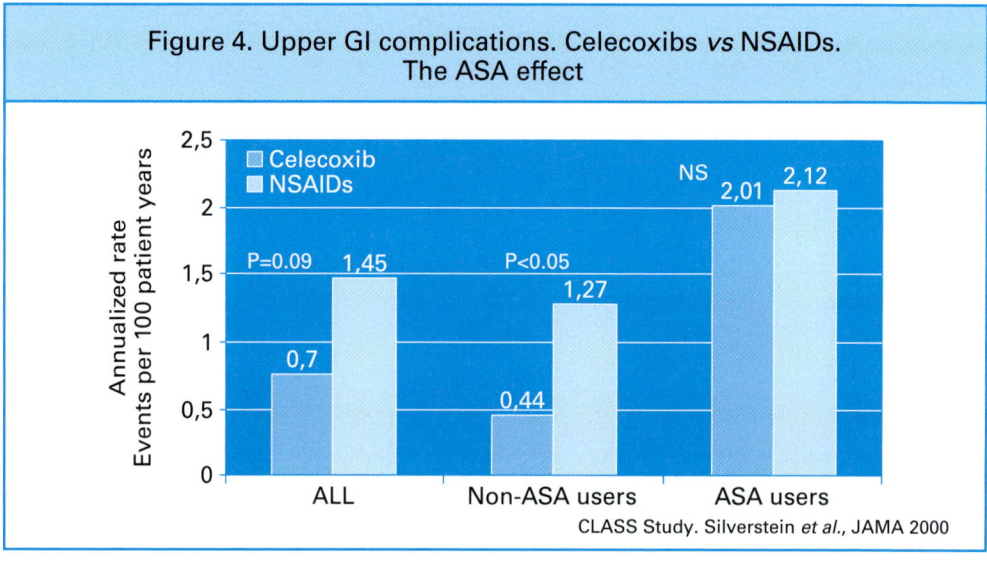

Figure 4. Upper GI complications. Celecoxibs *vs* NSAIDs. The ASA effect

CLASS Study. Silverstein *et al.*, JAMA 2000

Low-dose aspirin and the gastroduodenal tract

Low-dose aspirin induces acute mucosal damage in the gastroduodenal mucosa, although, as commented above, the clinical relevance of this is limited; 7% of patients taking low-dose aspirin also have chronic peptic ulcers and with almost no exception, all studies designed to evaluate the benefits of low-dose aspirin on vascular occlusive diseases have shown a significant increase in the incidence of GI bleeding. Based on the general population, early observational studies have reported risks of upper GI complications from 1 to 10 times higher among aspirin users, with an estimated pooled relative risk between 2 and 3.

Novel Developments in Gastroenterology.
P. Malfertheiner, L. Lundell, G. Tytgat, eds. John Libbey Eurotext, Paris © 2006, Addendum.

Chronic intestinal pseudo-obstruction syndrome

Olivier Goulet

Department of Pediatric, Gastroenterology Hepatology and Nutrition, National Reference Center for Rare Digestive Diseases, Hôpital Necker-Enfants Malades at the University of Paris René Descartes, France

Novel Developments in Gastroenterology.
P. Malfertheiner, L. Lundell, G. Tytgat, eds. John Libbey Eurotext, Paris © 2006, Addendum.

Chronic intestinal pseudo-obstruction syndrome

Olivier Goulet

Department of Pediatric, Gastroenterology Hepatology and Nutrition, National Reference Center for Rare Digestive Diseases, Hôpital Necker-Enfants Malades at the University of Paris René Descartes, France

The chronic intestinal pseudo-obstruction syndrome (CIPOS) is characterized by repetitive episodes or continuous symptoms and signs of bowel obstruction, including radiographic documentation of dilated bowel, in the absence of a fixed lumen occluding lesion [1, 2]. Most of the time, paediatricians deal with primary CIPOS, of which several histopathologic types and associated disorders have been described [3-12]. Regardless of the histologic type (myopathy or neuropathy), CIPOS always involves alterations of smooth muscle contractile function, leading to abnormal intestinal tract peristalsis and finally nutritional disorders from both intestinal failure and recurrent sepsis. Accompanying uropathies must be sought in all patients with CIPOS [13, 14]. Surveys of pediatric cases are published, including a large multicenter French study [15-17]. With adequate medico-surgical management, most pediatric patients with primary CIPOS now survive until adulthood.

Surgery for diagnosis

Variable clinical presentation and lack of specific diagnostic test may lead to surgery for diagnosis. Some patients, especially children and adolescents with an acute presentation, usually undergo exploratory laparotomy. In the absence of organic obstruction observed at laparotomy, a medico-surgical discussion is required for:

– performing intestinal full thickness biopsies at different levels for histopathologic analysis,
– performing an enterostomy according to the level of intestinal distension.

Such issues are controversial and we do consider that if the diagnosis of CIPOS is strongly suggested from the surgical exploration, careful biopsies shoud be performed. Regarding enterostomy, our experience tends to demonstrate that when it was not performed at first laparotomy, it will be done later on, thus increasing the risk of peritoneal adhesions.

Patients with evidence of CIPOS from clinical and radiological presentation should not be operated on to make the diagnosis. Patients who undergo laparotomy for enterostomy because of permanent or recurrent intestinal obstruction should have intestinal full thickness biopsies for specific diagnosis.

Medical treatment

Treatment is complex and very difficult to standardize. Despite the *in vitro* and *in vivo* pharmacological effects of different drugs, there is an inconsistency when translated into clinical setting for patients with CIPOS. During the acute phases of obstructive symptoms, nasogastric or, preferably, naso-duodenal succion, combined with intensive nursing (abdominal massages, intestinal catheterization), strict replacement of fluid losses and IV administration of prokinetic drugs allow transit to resume after a variable management duration. The placement of venting gastrostomy is of great benefit in avoiding the recurrent placement of nasogastric tubes. Percutaneous endoscopic gastrostomy tube (GT) placement is easily achieved. When surgery is required, a gastrostomy may be created during the same surgical procedure. Since enteral feeding should always be preferred to using parenteral nutrition (PN), intragastric administration of feeding may be achieved by the GT as continuous or bolus enteral feeding.

Enterostomy

In neonates and young infants, intestinal obstruction may last several weeks requiring total parenteral nutrition (TPN) with subsequent complications including catheter related sepsis and liver disease. Enterostomy may offer the chance to restart intestinal transit allowing feeding and reducing PN.

In some patients, attacks of intestinal obstruction are frequent or life threatening. Chronic bowel dilatation impairs intestinal motility creating a vicious circle which increases intra-luminal bacterial overgrowth with the subsequent risk of intestinal translocation, sepsis and liver disease. Enterostomy should be performed to bypass the functionnal obstruction and to obtain digestive decompression.

The location of enterostomy is a matter of debate. In case of obvious megacystis microcolon syndrome, a terminal ileostomy is required. However, we do recommend to perform a terminal ileostomy and to avoid colostomy whatever the clinical presentation and the histopathologic pattern. In our experience, all patients who underwent first colostomy were finally put on terminal ileostomy or jejnuostomy.

Outcome after ileostomy or jejunostomy varies according to the location of the enterostomy. Literature does not provide any evidence of a histopathology related prognosis. Less than 50% of patients improve after ileostomy by being weaned from PN. In our opinion, enterostomies (as distal as possible) are the most logical approach. Terminal ileostomy usually enables transit to resume and leads to a major long-term reduction in obstructive episodes. We currently perform an ileostomy to obtain durable intestinal autonomy without artificial nutrition, with the future plan to do a total or partial colectomy with ileorectal or colorectal pull-through [3].

Closure of the stoma

In children whom a decompression ileostomy has produced relief, but there is diffuse disease, the urge to re-establish connection with the defunctioned limb of the bowel should be resisted as this will only result in further episodes of obstruction [16]. In other words, performing an ileostomy and closing it because of clinical improvement results in the patient undergoing two surgical without resolution of the primary issues. This should be avoided. Conversely, in patients in which clear improvement from ileostomy is observed, with PN weaning and at least 2 years follow-up on enteral/oral feeding without exacerbations, total colectomy and ileorectal anastomosis with the Duhamel procedure may be considered. In our experience, two third of the patients who underwent this procedure remain off PN for long period of time if not definitive [3, 17].

Recurrent laparotomies

Patients with an enterostomy who continue to present with exacerbation of bowel obstruction are thought to have a mechanical obstruction. In the past, many children underwent multiple surgical procedures resulting in dense adhesions further aggravating obstruction. An excessive number of surgical procedures should be avoided. In a previous study, surgery was performed as a treatment 21 times with a mean of 3 procedures per patient [16]. This is similar to data reported, with 67 surgical procedures in 22 patients [6]. In the current largest study involving 105 pediatric infants and children, 71 patients underwent surgery during their illness, and 217 surgical procedures, a mean of 3 per patient, were performed [17]. Ostomy was the most performed procedure. Surgery may cause adhesions, so interpretations of subsequent obstructive episodes are difficult. Exploratory laparotomy for obstruction should be performed only when a clear mechanical obstruction has been demonstrated which remains very difficult to assess. Signs of peritonitis, extreme dilatation and pain in association with specific episode of obstruction points more towards a mechanical obstruction than functional obstruction and laparotomy may be required to relieve it.

Some patients, in whom there was no evidence of mechanical obstruction but segmented bowel dilatation, had improvement by placing a jejunostomy tube within a dilated loop. The use of this jejunostomy buttom device for daily intermittent bowel decompression was shown, in our experience, to improve bowel function allowing decreased PN intake. However, one should consider a child with three tubes: gastrostomy, jejunostomy and terminal ileostomy. Other authors proposed total enterectomy or segmental bowel resection [18-20].

Intestinal transplantation

In many cases of CIPOS, outcome is poor, with a constant risk of sepsis from intestinal bacterial overgrowth, and water-electrolytic disorders related to intraluminal fluid retention. Thus, intestinal transplantation (ITx) is the only definitive curative treatment especially when many medical and surgical attempts failed. ITx associated or not with liver transplantation is required in patients with primary neuro-muscular disease and PN related complications such as progressive or end stage liver disease or for those whose intravenous access has become unreliable and precarious because of repeated sepsis and extensive thrombosis. Transplant procedures vary according indication for liver transplant and based on the experience of the transplant surgical team [21-25]. Combined small bowel-liver transplantations or multivisceral transplantations including the stomach have been performed in refractory form of CIPOS associated with end stage liver disease [22-24]. Multivisceral transplantation (MVTx) was reported in 16 children at median age of 4 years [22]. Modified MVTx without the liver was performed in six patients. Actuarial patient survival for 1 year/2 years for period, I and II were 57.1%/42.9% and 88.9%/77.8%. None of the long-term survivors are on PN and all tolerate enteral feedings. Gastric emptying was substantially affected in one case. Bladder function did not improve in those with urinary retention problems. MVTx for CIPOS offers a lifesaving option with excellent function of the transplanted pancreas and stomach among survivors.

Ethical dilemnas may arise with children who will never be able to tolerate full enteral feeding. Some patients with severe CIPOS may be disabled because of chronic, massive GI dilatation refractory to stomal decompression or partial enterectomy. The poor quality of life might serve as indication for ITx, although usual criteria include progressive liver disease, the loss of vascular access, and absence recurring life-threatening sepsis.

In any case, patients and parents must be extensively informed about the risks of the procedure and about the outcome. Indeed in such patients in whom intestinal autonomy will never be achieved, intestinal transplantation may represent the logical therapy [26]. However, it is not yet established if the results of intestinal transplantation achieved with the motility disorders are equivalent to those experienced with other causes of intestinal failure. In themselves, the motility disorders present their own set of complicating factors, including determining the extent of the disease process (which may involve any part of the gastrointestinal tract), associated urological anomalies, and the type of organ transplantation required. Extensive workup and careful consideration is required before transplantation is undertaken. However, early referral is essential on initial presentation of complications for these patients to be provided optimal medical care ensuring transplantation an option. Multidisciplinary approach is mandatory [27].

References

1. Byrne WJ, Cipel L, Euler AR, *et al.* Chronic idiopathic intestinal pseudo-obstruction syndrome in children clinical characteristics and prognosis. *J Pediatr* 1977; 90: 585-9.
2. Rudolph CD, Hyman PE, Altschuler SM, *et al.* Diagnosis and treatment of chronic intestinal pseudo-obstruction in children: Report of consensus workshop. *J Pediatr Gastroenterol Nutr* 1997; 24: 102-12.
3. Goulet O, Jobert-Giraud A, Michel J-L, *et al.* Chronic intestinal pseudo-obstruction syndrome in pediatric patients. *Eur J Pediatr Surg* 1999; 9: 83-90.
4. Kern IB, Leece A, Bohane T. Congenital short gut, malrotation, and dysmotility of the small bowel. *J Pediatr Gastroenterol Nutr* 1990; 11: 411-5.
5. Ciftci AO, Cook RCM, Van Velzen D. Megacystic microcolon intestinal hypoperistalsis syndrome: evidence of a primary myocellular defect of contractile fiber synthesis. *J Pediatr Surg* 1996; 31: 1706-11.

6. Krishnamurthy S, Heng S, Schuffler M. Chronic intestinal pseudo-obstruction in infants and children caused by diverse abnormalities of myenteric plexus. *Gastroenterology* 1993; 104: 1398-408.
7. Gilbert J, Ibdah JA. Intestinal pseudo-obstruction as a manifestation of impaired mitochondrial fatty acid oxidation. *Med Hypotheses* 2005; 64: 586-9.
8. Kohler M, Pease PW, Upadhyay V. Megacystis-microcolon-intestinal hypoperistalsis syndrome in siblings: case report and review of the literature. *Eur J Pediatr Surg* 2004; 14: 362-7.
9. De Giorgio R, Sarnelli G, Corinaldesi R, Stanghellini V. Advances in our understanding of the pathology of chronic intestinal pseudo-obstruction. *Gut* 2004; 53: 1549-52.
10. Wedel T, Tafazzoli K, Sollner S, Krammer HJ, Aring C, Holschneider AM. Mitochondrial myopathy (complex I deficiency) associated with chronic intestinal pseudo-obstruction. *Eur J Pediatr Surg* 2003; 13: 201-5.
11. Feldstein AE, Miller SM, El-Youssef M, *et al*. Chronic intestinal pseudoobstruction associated with altered interstitial cells of cajal networks. *J Pediatr Gastroenterol Nutr* 2003; 36: 492-7.
12. Wedel T, Tafazzoli K, Sollner S, Krammer HJ, Aring C, Holschneider AM. Mitochondrial myopathy (complex I deficiency) associated with chronic intestinal pseudo-obstruction. *Eur J Pediatr Surg* 2003; 13: 201-5.
13. Schuffler MD, Pagon RA, Schwartz R, Bill AH. Visceral myopathy of the gastrointestinal and genitourinary racts in infants. *Gastroenterology* 1988; 94: 892-8.
14. Lapointe SP, Rivet C, Goulet O, Fekete CN, Lortat-Jacob S. Urological manifestations associated with chronic intestinal pseudo-obstructions in children. *J Urol* 2002; 168: 1768-70.
15. Vargas J, Sachs P, Ament ME. Chronic intestinal pseudo-obstruction syndrome in pediatrics. Results of a national survey by members of the NASPGN. *J Pediatr Gastroenterol Nutr* 1988; 7: 323-32.
16. Nonaka M, Goulet O, Arhan P, *et al.* Primary intestinal myopathy, a cause of chronic intestinal pseudo-obstruction syndrome. *Pediatr Pathol* 1989; 9: 409-24.
17. Faure C, Goulet O, Ategbo S, *et al.* Chronic intestinal pseudoobstruction syndrome. Clinical analysis, Outcome, and prognosis in 105 children. *Dig Dis Sci* 1999; 44: 953-9.
18. Mughal MM, Irving MH. Treatment of end stage chronic intestinal pseudo-obstruction by subtotal enterectomy and home parenteral nutrition. *Gut* 1988; 29: 1613-7.
19. Nayci A, Avlan D, Polat A, Aksoyek S. Treatment of intestinal pseudo obstruction by segmental resection. *Pediatr Surg Int* 2003; 19: 44-6.
20. Shibata C, Naito H, Funayama Y, *et al.* Surgical treatment of chronic intestinal pseudo-obstruction: report of three cases. *Surg Today* 2003; 33: 58-61.
21. Goulet O, Lacaille F, Jan D, Ricour C. Intestinal transplantation: indications, results and strategy. *Curr Opin Clin Nutr Metab Care* 2000; 3: 329-38.
22. Loinaz C, Mittal N, Kato T, Miller B, Rodriguez M, Tzakis A. Multivisceral transplantation for pediatric intestinal pseudo-obstruction: single center's experience of 16 cases. *Transplant Proc* 2004; 36: 312-3.
23. Masetti M, Di Benedetto F, Cautero N, *et al.* Intestinal transplantation for chronic intestinal pseudo-obstruction in adult patients. *Am J Transplant* 2004; 4: 286-92.
24. Bond GJ, Reyes JD. Intestinal transplantation for total/near-total aganglionosis and intestinal pseudo-obstruction. *Semin Pediatr Surg* 2004; 13: 286-92.
25. Grant D, Abu-Elmagd K, Reyes J, Tzakis A, Langnas A, Fishbein T, Goulet O, Farmer D, on behalf of the Intestine Transplant Registry. 2003 report of the intestine transplant registry: a new era has dawned. *Ann Surg* 2005; 241: 607-13.
26. Goulet O, Ruemmele F. Causes and management of intestinal failure in children. *Gastroenterology* 2006; 130: S16-28.
27. Chronic idiopathic intestinal pseudo-obstruction: the need for a multidisciplinary approach to management. *Proc Nutr Soc* 2004; 63: 473-80.

Although the recommended prophylactic doses of aspirin are now lower (75-300 mg/day) than several years ago, current data suggest that even the lower doses are still toxic to the GI tract. The combination of the results from nine studies where aspirin was used from a range of 75-325 mg daily showed that the monthly probability of GI bleeding per 1,000 patients ranged between 0 and 2.1. In another recent meta-analysis of 24 randomized controlled trials of aspirin prescribed for vascular occlusive diseases, where the average treatment duration was at least 28 months, GI bleeding occurred in 2.30% of patients taking low-dose aspirin (50-162.5 mg/day) and 1.45% taking placebo In clinical practice, outside clinical trials, in unselected patients discharged from hospital taking low-dose aspirin and with a mean follow-up of 45 months, the reported incidence of major upper GI bleeding events was 1.2 events per 100 patients-years.

Selected references

- Bombardier C, Laine L, Reicin A, Shapiro D, Burgos-Vargas R, Davis B, *et al.* Comparison of upper gastrointestinal toxicity of rofecoxib and naproxen in patients with rheumatoid arthritis. VIGOR Study Group. *N Engl J Med* 2000; 343 (21): 1520-8.
- Chan FK, Chung SC, Suen BY, Lee YT, Leung WK, Leung VK, *et al.* Preventing recurrent upper gastrointestinal bleeding in patients with Helicobacter pylori infection who are taking low-dose aspirin or naproxen. *N Engl J Med* 2001; 344: 967-73.
- Emery P, Zeidler H, Kvien TK, Guslandi M, Naudin R, Stead H, *et al.* Celecoxib *versus* diclofenac in long-term management of rheumatoid arthritis: randomised double-blind comparison. *Lancet* 1999; 354: 2106-111.
- Hawkey CJ. Nonsteroidal anti-inflammatory drug gastropathy. *Gastroenterology* 2000; 119 (2): 521-35.
- Laine L, Harper S, Simon T, Bath R, Johanson J, Schwartz H, *et al.* A randomized trial comparing the effect of rofecoxib, a cylooxigenase 2-specific inhibitor, with that of ibuprofen on the gastroduodenal mucosa of patients with osteoarthritis. *Gastroenterology* 1999; 117: 776-83.
- Lanas A, Bajador E, Serrano P, Fuentes J, Carreño S, Guardia J, *et al.* Nitrovasodilators, low-dose aspirin, nonsteroidal anti-inflammatory drugs, and the risk of upper gastrointestinal bleeding. *N Engl J Med* 2000; 343: 834-9.
- Lanas A, Perez-Aisa MA, Feu F, Ponce J, Saperas E, Santolaria S, Rodrigo L, Balanzo J, Bajador E, Almela P, Navarro JM, Carballo F, Castro M, Quintero E; Investigators of the Asociacion Espanola de Gastroenterologia (AEG). A nationwide study of mortality associated with hospital admission due to severe gastrointestinal events and those associated with non-steroidal anti-inflammatory drug use. *Am J Gastroenterol* 2005; 100: 1685-93.
- Rostom A, Dube C, Wells G, Tugwell P, Welch V, Jolicœur E, *et al.* Prevention of NSAID-induced gastroduodenal ulcers. *Cochrane Database Syst Rev* 2004; (4 (CD002296)): 1-111.
- Schnitzer TJ, Burmester GR, Mysler E, Hochberg MC, Doherty M, Ehrsam E, *et al.* Comparison of lumiracoxib with naproxen and ibuprofen in the Therapeutic Arthritis Research and Gastrointestinal Event Trial (TARGET), reduction in ulcer complications: randomised controlled trial. *Lancet* 2004; 364 (9435): 665-74.
- Silverstein FE, Faich G, Goldstein JL, Simon LS, Pincus T, Whelton A, *et al.* Gastrointestinal toxicity with celecoxib *vs* nonsteroidal anti-inflammatory drugs for osteoarthritis and rheumatoid arthritis: the CLASS study: A randomized controlled trial. Celecoxib Long-term Arthritis Safety Study. *JAMA* 2000; 284 (10): 1247-55.
- Singh G, Fort JG, Goldstein JL, Levy RA, Hanrahan PS, Bello AE, *et al.* Celecoxib *versus* naproxen and diclofenac in osteoarthritis patients: SUCCESS-I Study. *Am J Med* 2006; 119 (3): 255-66.

- Tramer MR, Moore RA, Reynolds DJ, McQuay HJ. Quantitative estimation of rare adverse events which follow a biological progression: a new model applied to chronic NSAID use. *Pain* 2000; 85 (1-2): 169-82.
- Wolfe MM, Lichtenstein DR, Singh G. Gastrointestinal toxicity of nonsteroidal antiinflammatory drugs. *N Engl J Med* 1999; 340: 1888-99.

Drug-induced small/large bowel injury

Christoph Beglinger

Division of Gastroenterology, University Hospital of Basel, Switzerland

Nonsteroidal anti-inflammatory drugs (NSAIDs) are among the most frequently used drugs in the world. They are primarily prescribed to manage pain and inflammation associated with osteoarthritis or rheumatoid arthritis [1]. In addition, aspirin is used for prophylaxis of cardiovascular disease. Seventy percent of people 65 years or older take NSAIDs including aspirin at least once weekly and 34% need at least one pill every day [2]. In the 1960s, NSAIDs were developed as a potentially safe alternative to aspirin, which is associated with significant gastrointestinal side effects [3]. However, NSAID-induced gastrointestinal toxicity is among the most common drug-related serious adverse events and thus, the goal of a safer aspirin has not been achieved. Moreover, NSAID-associated GI complications appear to increase annually and are currently responsible for 5-10 billion dollars in hospitalisation charges and lost work time [4]. The availability of a new generation of safer NSAIDs is therefore of crucial clinical relevance.

Cyclooxygenase (COX) is the rate-limiting enzyme for the metabolic conversion of arachidonic acid to prostaglandins and related eicanosids. Cyclooxygenase exists in at least two isoforms, COX-1 and COX-2, which are both inhibited by non-selective NSAIDs. COX-1 is constitutively expressed in most tissues and cell types and is the predominant isoenzyme in the normal gastric mucosa. COX-1-mediated prostaglandin synthesis plays an important role in maintaining gastrointestinal mucosal protection [1]. In contrast, COX-2 is primarily an inducible enzyme, which is believed to generate prostaglandins mediating inflammation and pain throughout the body. The anti-inflammatory effects of non-selective NSAIDs seem to be the consequence of COX-2 inhibition, whereas the adverse effects in the GI tract are believed to occur primarily *via* inhibition of COX-1 [5].

The development of COX-2-selective inhibitors (Coxibs) such as celecoxib, lumiracoxib or valdecoxib offers the promise of relieving pain and inflammation without any effect on COX-1 and its cytoprotective function [6]. Within the first three months of its availability, celecoxib became the fastest selling drug in history [7].

The current review will focus on the differences of non-selective NSAIDs and COX-2-specific inhibitors with respect to the incidence of dyspeptic symptoms, erosions, endoscopic ulcers and ulcer complications (bleeding, obstruction, perforation) as well as their current clinical application. In addition, we will discuss the effects of traditional NSAIDs and COX-2 inhibitors on the gut, as well as their role in chemoprevention.

Gastrointestinal risks of non-selective NSAIDs

NSAID-associated serious adverse events result in 107,000 hospitalisations and 16,500 deaths per year in the United States [8]. Data from the Tennessee Medicaid Program suggest that there are 1.25 excess hospitalisations per 100 patient-years in regular NSAID users [8, 9]. In the United Kingdom, aspirin and non-aspirin NSAIDs cause approximately 3,500 hospitalisations and 400 deaths from ulcer bleeding per year in patients 60 years and older [10, 11].

NSAID use increases the risk of gastrointestinal complications 2-6 times [12, 13]. The risk of NSAID-associated GI complications is basically the consequence of three mechanisms (1) platelet dysfunction in the presence of underlying lesions, (2) exacerbation of pre-existing ulcers and (3) induction of new ulcers by NSAIDs [14]. Epidemiological studies have demonstrated that the use of NSAIDs increases the risk of GI adverse events-related death (OR 4.79-7.62), peptic ulcer bleeding (OR 3.09-4.5), hospitalisations (OR 3.9.-5.5) and surgery (OR 7.75) [15].

Effects of NSAIDs on the gut

As many as 70% of patients taking regularly NSAIDs develop asymptomatic small intestinal inflammation, which may lead to iron deficiency, blood loss and hypoalbuminaemia [16]. Further complications of chronic NSAID use are (1) ulcers of the small and large intestine, which may bleed or perforate, (2) ileal dysfunction, (3) diaphragmatic small intestinal strictures, which may cause obstruction, (4) colitis, which may led to bloody diarrhoea and (5) NSAID enteropathy, which may result in chronic blood loss [16-23].

Increased permeability is believed to be a prerequisite for the development of NSAID-induced enteropathy [24]. An enhanced permeability may expose the mucosa to luminal toxins and enable bacterial invasion of the intestinal mucosa [16, 25]. The mechanisms, by which NSAIDs enhance intestinal permeability, are unknown, but may be related to a reduction of endogenous intestinal mucosal prostaglandins and/or interference with mitochondrial energy metabolism [26]. The relevance of mucosal prostaglandin depletion is supported by the observation, that administration of exogenous prostaglandins attenuates NSAID-induced, enhanced intestinal permeability.

Data from epidemiological studies suggest, that NSAIDs increase the risk of lower gastrointestinal complications including bleeding, perforation, obstruction, ulcerations, and symptomatic diverticular disease [16, 17, 20, 27, 28]. Just recently, Laine *et al.* published the post hoc analysis of a large prospective, double blind outcome study of rofecoxib *versus* naproxen to assess the risk of serious lower GI clinical events [29]. In this study, naproxen treated patients had an annualised incidence of 0.9% lower GI complications, which accounted for approximately 40% of all serious GI events [29].

The mechanisms of NSAID-induced lower GI events are uncertain. A direct effect of NSAIDs on enterocytes has been suggested by Bjarnason [16]. More recent studies provide evidence for the hypothesis that inhibition of COX-1 and COX-2- mediated prostaglandin synthesis may be responsible for NSAID-induced intestinal damage. The latter concept is in line with the observation, that in patients with anaemia caused by NSAID enteropathy, misoprostol led to a significant increase of haemoglobin level [30].

Effects of COX-2 inhibitors on the gut

Hunt *et al.* examined gastrointestinal micro bleeding before and after treatment with ibuprofen (2,400 mg daily), rofecoxib (25 and 50 mg) or placebo in healthy subjects [31]. Blood loss was measured using ^{51}Cr labelled red blood cells. Faecal red blood cell loss was significantly higher with ibuprofen than with rofecoxib or placebo. Both doses of rofecoxib were statistically not different from placebo [31].

The effect of COX-2 inhibitors on lower GI events was assessed in the study of Laine *et al.* including 8076 rheumatoid arthritis patients, who randomly received naproxen 500 mg twice daily or rofecoxib 50 mg daily [29]. Serious lower GI clinical events were defined as bleeding with a 2g/dl drop in haemoglobin or hospitalisation for perforation, obstruction, ulceration or diverticulitis. The authors found that rofecoxib was associated with a 54% lower risk of serious lower GI events compared to naproxen. 208 patients would need to be treated with rofecoxib instead of naproxen to avert 1 serious lower GI event [29].

References

1. Goldstein JL, Correa P, Zhao WW, Burr AM, Hubbard RC, Verburg KM, Geis GS. Reduced incidence of gastroduodenal ulcers with celecoxib, a novel cyclooxygenase-2 inhibitor, compared to naproxen in patients with arthritis. *Am J Gastroenterol* 2001; 96: 1019-27.
2. Talley NJ, Evans JM, Fleming KC, Harmsen WS, Zinsmeister AR, Melton JL. Nonsteroidal anti-inflammatory drugs and dyspepsia in the elderly. *Dig Dis Sci* 1995; 40: 1345-50.
3. James MW, Hawkey CJ. Assessment of non-steroidal anti-inflammatory drug (NSAID) damage in the human gastrointestinal tract. *Br J Clin Pharmacol* 2003; 56: 146-55.
4. Lichtenberger LM. Where is the evidence that cyclooxygenase inhibition is the primary cause of nonsteroidal anti-inflammatory drug (NSAID)-induced gastrointestinal injury? Topical injury revisited. *Biochem Pharmacol* 2001; 61: 631-7.

5. Laine L, Harper S, Simon T, Bath R, Johanson J, Schwartz H, Stern S, Quan H, Bolognese J. A randomized trial comparing the effect of rofecoxib, a cyclooxygenase 2-specific inhibitor, with that of ibuprofen on the gastroduodenal mucosa of patients with osteoarthritis. Rofecoxib Osteoarthritis Endoscopy Study Group. *Gastroenterology* 1999; 117: 776-83.
6. Bombardier C. An evidence-based evaluation of the gastrointestinal safety of coxibs. *Am J Cardiol* 2002; 89 (S): 3D-9D.
7. Mamdani M, Rochon PA, Juurlink DN, Kopp A, Anderson GM, Naglie G, Austin PC, Laupacis A. Observational study of upper gastrointestinal haemorrhage in elderly patients given selective cyclooxygenase-2 inhibitors or conventional non-steroidal anti-inflammatory drugs. *Br Med J* 2002; 325: 624-9.
8. Wolfe MM, Lichtenstein DR, Singh G. Gastrointestinal toxicity of nonsteroidal antiinflammatory drugs. *N Engl J Med* 1999; 340: 1888-99.
9. Singh G. Recent considerations in nonsteroidal anti-inflammatory drug gastropathy. *Am J Med* 1998; 105: 31S-38S.
10. Langman MJ. Ulcer complications associated with anti-inflammatory drug use. What is the extent of the disease burden? *Pharmacoepidemiol Drug Saf* 2001; 10: 13-9.
11. Hawkey CJ, Langman MJ. Non-steroidal anti-inflammatory drugs: overall risks and management. Complementary roles fo COX-2 inhibitors and proton pump inhibitors. *Gut* 2003; 52: 600-8.
12. Laine L. Gastrointestinal effects of NSAIDs and coxibs. *J Pain Symptom Manage* 2003; 25S: S32-S40.
13. Hernandez-Diaz S, Rodriguez LA. Association between nonsteroidal anti-inflammatory drugs and upper gastrointestinal tract bleeding/perforation: an overview of epidemiologic studies published in the 1990s. *Arch Intern Med* 2000; 160: 2093-9.
14. McCarthy DM. Prevention and treatment of gastrointestinal symptoms and complications due to NSAIDs. *Best Pract Res Clin Gastroenterol* 2001; 15: 755-73.
15. Hunt RH. Motion-Cyclo-oxygenase-2 selective nonsteroidal anti-inflammatory drugs are as safe as placebo for the stomach: arguments for the motion. *Can J Gastroenterol* 2003; 17: 339-41.
16. Bjarnason I, Hayllar J, MacPherson AJ, Russell AS. Side effects of nonsteroidal anti-inflammatory drugs on the small and large intestine in humans. *Gastroenterology* 1993; 104: 1832-47.
17. Allison MC, Howatson AG, Torrance CJ, Lee FD, Russell RI. Gastrointestinal damage associated with the use of nonsteroidal antiinflammatory drugs. *N Engl J Med* 1992; 327: 749-54.
18. Bjarnason I, Williams P, So A, Zanelli GD, Levi AJ, Gumpel JM, *et al.* Intestinal permeability and inflammation in rheumatoid arthritis: effects of non-steroidal anti-inflammatory drugs. *Lancet* 1984; 2: 1171-4.
19. Bjarnason I, Zanelli G, Smith T, Prouse P, Williams P, Smethurst P, *et al.* Nonsteroidal antiinflammatory drug-induced intestinal inflammation in humans. *Gastroenterology* 1987; 93: 480-9.
20. Bjarnason I, Zanelli G, Prouse P, Smethurst P, Smith T, Levi S, *et al.* Blood and protein loss *via* small-intestinal inflammation induced by non-steroidal anti-inflammatory drugs. *Lancet* 1987; 2: 711-4.
21. Bjarnason I, Price AB, Zanelli G, Smethurst P, Burke M, Gumpel JM, *et al.* Clinicopathological features of nonsteroidal anti-inflammatory drug-induced small intestinal strictures. *Gastroenterology* 1988: 94: 1070-4.
22. Segal AW, Isenberg DA, Hajirousou V, Tolfree S, Clark J, Snaith ML. Preliminary evidence for gut involvement in the pathogenesis of rheumatoid arthritis? *Br J Rheumatol* 1986; 25: 162-6.
23. Lanas A, Serrano P, Bajador E, Esteva F, Benito R, Sainz R. Evidence of aspirin use in both upper and lower gastrointestinal perforation. *Gastroenterology* 1997; 112: 683-9.
24. Sigthorsson G, Crane R, Simon T, Hoover M, Quan H, Bolognese J, Bjarnason I. COX-2 inhibition with rofecoxib does not increase intestinal permeability in healthy subjects: a double blind crossover study comparing rofecoxib with placebo and indomethacin. *Gut* 2000; 47: 527-32.

25. Bjarnason I, Fehilly B, Smethurst P, Menzies IS, Levi AJ. Importance of local versus systemic effects of non-steroidal anti-inflammatory drugs in increasing small intestinal permeability in man. *Gut* 1991; 32: 275-7.
26. Somasundaram S, Hayllar H, Rafi S, Wrigglesworth JM, Macpherson AJ, Bjarnason I. The biochemical basis of non-steroidal anti-inflammatory drug-induced damage to the gastrointestinal tract: a review and a hypothesis. *Scand J Gastroenterol* 1995; 30: 289-99.
27. Langman MJS, Morgan L, Worrall A. Use of anti-inflammatory drugs by patients admitted with small or large bowel perforations and haemorrhage. *Br Med J* 1985; 290: 347-9.
28. Wilcox CM, Alexander LN, Cotsonis GA, Clark WS. Nonsteroidal antiinflammatory drugs are associated with both upper and lower gastrointestinal bleeding. *Dig Dis Sci* 1997; 42: 990-7.
29. Laine L, Connors LG, Reicin A, Hawkey CJ, Burgos-Vargas R, Schnitzer TJ, Yu Q, Bombardier C. Serious lower gastrointestinal clinical events with nonselective NSAID or coxib use. *Gastroenterology* 2003; 124: 288-92.
30. Morris AJ, Murray L, Sturrock RD, Madhok R, Capell HA, Mackenzie JF. Short report: the effect of misoprostol on the anaemia of NSAID enteropathy. *Aliment Pharmacol Ther* 1994; 8: 343-6.
31. Hunt RH, Bowen B, James C, *et al.* COX-2 specific inhibition with MK-096 25 or 50 mg Q.D. over 4 weeks does not increase fecal blood loss. A controlled study with placebo and ibuprofen 800 mg T.I.D. *Am J Gastroenterol* 1998; 93: 1671.

Prevention of mucosal injury: whom, when, and how?

Jaroslaw Regula

Department of Gastroenterology, Institute of Oncology, Warsaw, Poland

Oesophageal injury

Drug-induced injury should be prevented mainly in elderly patients, with co-morbidities, who are bedridden and in whom oesophageal peristalsis is impaired. Long list of drugs that are known to induce oesophageal injury include: alendronate, potassium, non-steroidal antinflammatory drugs (NSAIDs), quinidine, tetracycline, clindamycine, ferrous compounds and others. People treated with these substances should be warned about possible damage and advised to modify their habits. These include: drinking lots of water and avoiding horizontal and semi horizontal position for at least half hour after ingestion of these drugs. Proton pump inhibitors can be used in selected cases to diminish additional damage caused by gastric refluxate.

Gastroduodenal injury

Gastroduodenal drug-injury is most often caused by NSAIDs. Current data are not sufficient to recommend adequate preventive measures with confidence. Recent studies on COX-2 inhibitors cardiovascular complications caused great uncertainty and consternation. Moreover, it seems that similar cardiovascular complications can also be attributed to most of classical NSAIDs [1]. Classical NSAIDs have never been studied properly using current methodology similar to large COX-2 trials.

The factors increasing the risk of gastroduodenal injury in patients using NSAID are presented in *Figure 1*. Patients fulfilling at least one of the listed risk factors should be offered gastroduodenal prophylaxis while on NSAIDs. Avoidance of NSAIDs especially in patients with cardiovascular risk, replacing them with acetaminophen or drugs from

> **Figure 1. Risk factors for NSAID-associated gastrointestinal complications**
>
> - Personal history of complicated ulcer disease
> - Concurrent use of more than 1 NSAID (including aspirin)
> - Use of high NSAID doses
> - Concurrent use of an anticoagulant
> - Personal history of uncomplicated ulcer disease
> - Advanced age
> - Concurrent use of steroids
>
> Scheiman, 2006

other therapeutic groups is still the best prevention. If avoidance of NSAID is not possible, the smallest possible dose should be used. Gastroduodenal prophylaxis is not necessary only in the absence risk factors. In all other patients the most popular and practically advisable prophylaxis is the concurrent usage of proton pump inhibitors (PPI). Two recent studies suggest that similar prophylactic effect may be obtained with 20 and 40 mg of esomeprazole [2] as well as with 20 mg and 40 mg of pantoprazole [3]. Therefore, smaller of the two studied doses of the above PPI may be recommended. Other PPIs share similar features. Misoprostol as concurrent prophylactic drug could also be recommended; prevention of serious NSAIDs complications was documented long time ago [4]. However, frequent side effects of misoprostol and poorer tolerance than PPIs decrease the practicality of this drug.

Replacement of classical NSAIDs by COX-2 inhibitors was a strong option until recently. COX-2 inhibitors decrease the risk of gastroduodenal damage by roughly 50% [5, 6]. Degree of prevention of COX-2 therapy is similar to concurrent classical NSAID plus PPI [7]. However, the price to pay is the increased risk of cardiovascular complications including myocardial infarction and death [8, 9]. Additionally, low dose aspirin administered as cardiovascular prevention ruins all gastroduodenal benfits of COX-2 inhibitors [6, 10].

Low dose aspirin is also responsible for gastroduodenal damage and preventive measures should be similar to those of classical NSAIDs; concurrent proton pump inhibitors is the preferred option. Additional beneficial effect of *Helicobacter pylori* eradication is well documented in this subgroup of patients [11]. Replacement of aspirin (plus PPI) by clopidogrel alone is not justified [12].

In patients with the highest risk of gastroduodenal damage (multiple risk factors) COX-2 inhibitors plus proton pump inhibitors should be considered because PPI decrease ulcer risk not only in classical NSAID but also in COX-2 users [13]. Suggestions concerning preventive measures in patients requiring prolonged NSAID therapy is shown in *Figure 2*.

Figure 2. Choice of NSAID in patients with gastrointestinal (GI) and/or cardiovascular (CV) risk factors

	No CV risk	With CV risk (usually using aspirin)
No GI risk	NSAID	NSAID
Intermediate GI risk	NSAID or coxib with PPI or misoprostol	NSAID with PPI or misoprostol
High GI risk	Coxib or NSAID with PPI	PPI (if on aspirin)

Small/large bowel injury

The knowledge about the NSAID injury of the intestines and its prevention is much smaller as compared to gastroduodenal damage. Unfortunately, small and large bowel injury is not prevented by concurrent use of proton pump inhibitors. Several options have been tried in experimental studies and small clinical trials including concurrent prostaglandins, metronidazole, sulfasalazine, or fish oil administration with conflicting results. Obviously, COX-2 inhibitors appear to be safer to the small intestine than traditional NSAIDs as shown in recent studies using capsule endoscopy technology [14]. However, the practical approach to small/large bowel injury in patients requiring NSAID therapy has yet to be elucidated in high quality clinical trials.

References

1. Kearney PM, Baigent C, Godwin J, *et al.* Do selective cyclo-oxygenase-2 inhibitors and traditional non-steroidal anti-inflammatory drugs increase the risk of atheromathosis? Meta-analysis of randomized trials. *Br Med J* 2006; 332: 1302.
2. Hawkey C, Talley NJ, Yeomans ND, *et al.* Improvements with esomeprazole in patients with upper gastrointestinal symptoms taking non-steroidal antiinflammatory drugs, including selective COX-2 inhibitors. *Am J Gastroenterol* 2005; 100: 1028-36.
3. Regula J, Butruk E, Dekkers CPM, *et al.* Prevention of NSAID-associated gastrointestinal lesions: a comparison study pantoprazole versus omeprazole. *Am J Gastroenterol* 2006; 101: 1747-55.

4. Silverstein FE, Graham DY, Senior Jr, *et al.* Misoprostol reduces serious gastrointestinal complications in patients with rheumatoid arthritis receiving nonsteroidal anti-inflammatory drugs. A randomized, double-blind, placebo controlled trial. *Ann Int Med* 1995; 123: 241-9.
5. Bombardier C, Laine L, Reicin A, *et al.* Comparison of upper gastrointestinal toxicity of rofecoxib and naproxen in patients with rheumatoid arthritis. VIGOR study group. *N Engl J Med* 2000; 343: 1520-8.
6. Silverstein FE, Faich G, Goldstein JL, *et al.* Gastrointestinal toxicity with celecoxib vs nonsteroidal anti-inflammatory drugs for osteoarthritis and rheumatoid arthritis: the CLASS study: a randomized controlled trial. Celecoxib long-term arthritis safety study. *JAMA* 2000; 284: 1247-55.
7. Chan FK, Hung LC, Suen BY, *et al.* Celecoxib versus diclofenac and omeprazole in reducing the risk of recurrent ulcer bleeding in patients with arthritis. *N Engl J Med* 2002; 347: 2104-10.
8. Bresalier RS, Sandler RS, Quan H, *et al.* Cardiovascular events associated with rofecoxib in a colorectal adenoma chemoprevention trial. *N Engl J Med* 2005; 352: 1092-102.
9. Solomon SD, McMurray JJV, Pfeffer MS, *et al.* for the Adenoma Prevention with Celecoxib (APC) study investigators. Cardiovascular risk associated with celecoxib in a clinical trial for colorectal adenoma prevention. *N Engl J Med* 2005: 352: 1071-80.
10. Laine L, Maller ES, Yu C, *et al.* Ulcer formation with low-dose enteric coated aspirin and the effect of COX-2 selective inhibition: a double-blind trial. *Gastroenterology* 2004; 127: 395-402.
11. Lai KC, Lam SK, Chu KM, *et al.* Lansoprazole for the prevention of recurrences of ulcer complications from long-term low-dose aspirin use. *N Engl J Med* 2002; 346: 2033-8.
12. Chan FKL, Ching JyL, Hung LCT, *et al.* Clopidogrel versus aspririn and esomeprazole to prevent recurrent ulcer bleeding. *N Engl J Med* 2005; 238: 352-3.
13. Scheiman JM, Yeomans ND, Talley NJ, *et al.* Prevention of ulcers by esomeprazole in at-risk patients using non-selective NSAIDs and COX-2 inhibitors. *Am J Gastroenterol* 2006; 101: 701-10.
14. Goldstein JL, *et al.* Video capsule endoscopy to prospectively assess small bowel injury with celecoxib, naproxen plus omeprazole, and placebo. *Clin Gastroenterol Hepatol* 2005; 3: 133-41.

Role of endoscopy in diagnosis and therapy of drug-induced UGI bleeding

Joseph Sung

Center for Emerging Infectious Diseases, Faculty of Medicine, The Chinese University of Hong-Kong

In a recent case-control study to determine the risk of peptic ulcer UGIB associated with coxibs, NSAID and aspirin, Lanas *et al.* reported that non-aspirin-NSAID use increased the risk of UGIB (RR: 5.3;95%CI 4.5-6.2). Rofecoxib therapy increased the risk of UGIB (RR: 2.1;1.1-4.0), whereas celecoxib, paracetamol or concomitant use of a PPI with an NSAID presented no increased risk. Non-aspirin antiplatelet therapy (clopidogrel/ticlopidine) had a similar risk of UGIB (RR: 2.8;1.9-4.2) to cardioprotective aspirin at a dose of 100 mg/daily (RR: 2.7;2.0-3.6) or anticoagulants (RR:2.8;2.1-3.7). There was an apparent interaction between low-dose aspirin and use of either non-aspirin-NSAIDs, coxibs or thienopyridines which increased further the risk of UGIB in a similar way. These ulcers are usually bigger, deeper, multiple and more difficult to treat because of bleeding diathesis associated.

Endoscopy offers an accurate diagnosis, assessment of risk and therapy. Early endoscopy is recommended but how early? In a recent study comparing early endoscopy (within 24 hours) *versus* "very early" endoscopy (within 6 hours), no significant advantage has been shown in the latter approach.

Endoscopic hemostasis includes injection, thermocoagulation and mechanical hemostasis. A recent meta-analysis show that, when epinephrine is used, addition of a second therapy is necessary. Combining injection with another modality will reduce recurrent bleeding, surgery rate and mortality.

There are controversies on the management of a large ulcer with adherent blood clot. Would medical therapy alone without endoscopic treatment be justified? A randomized study comparing the use of PPI alone *versus* combination of PPI with endoscopic therapy showed that endoscopic treatment is still necessary to prevent recurrent bleeding.

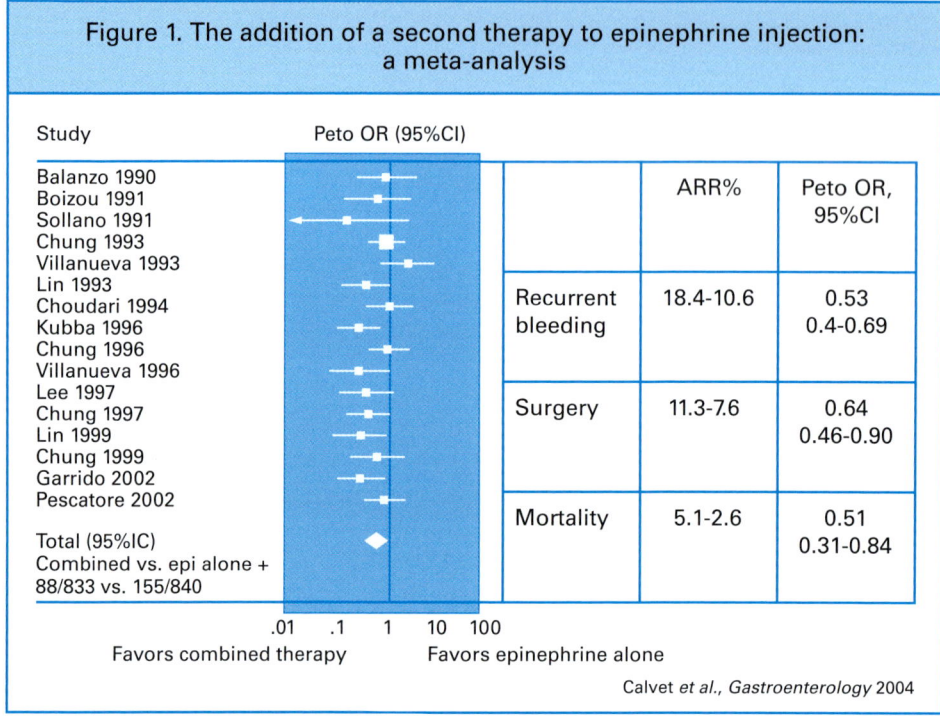

Figure 1. The addition of a second therapy to epinephrine injection: a meta-analysis

Calvet et al., Gastroenterology 2004

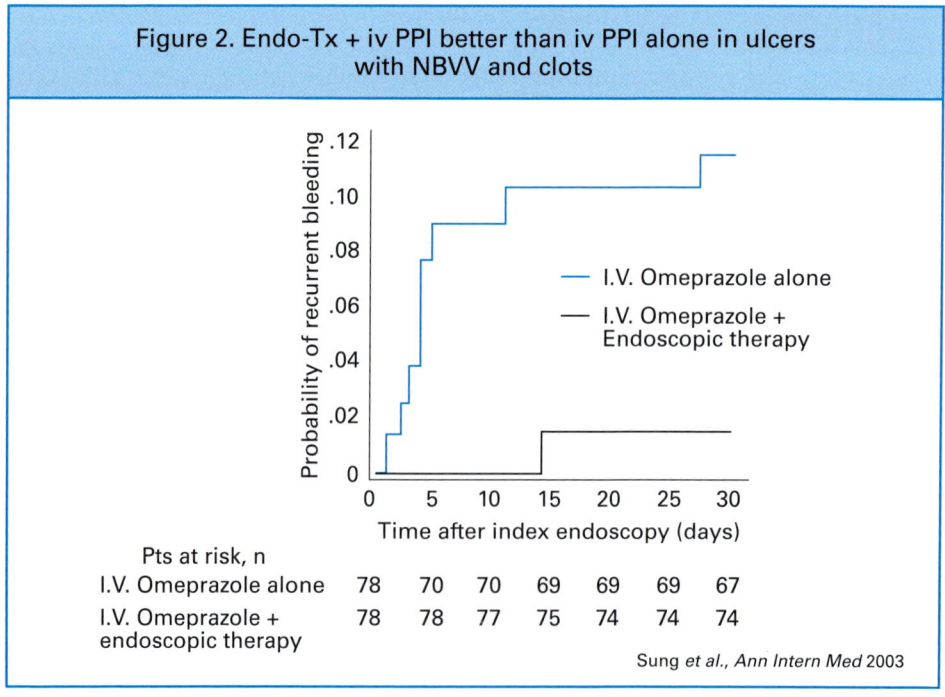

Figure 2. Endo-Tx + iv PPI better than iv PPI alone in ulcers with NBVV and clots

Sung et al., Ann Intern Med 2003

There are some suggestions that a scheduled 2nd look endoscopy on the next day after the index bleeding and endoscopic therapy would benefit the patient by reducing further rebleeding. In a recent randomized study comparing the use of PPI and scheduled 2nd endoscopy, rebleeding rate was found to be comparable with the two approaches. Therefore, when high dose PPI is given, a routine 2nd look endoscopy is not justified.

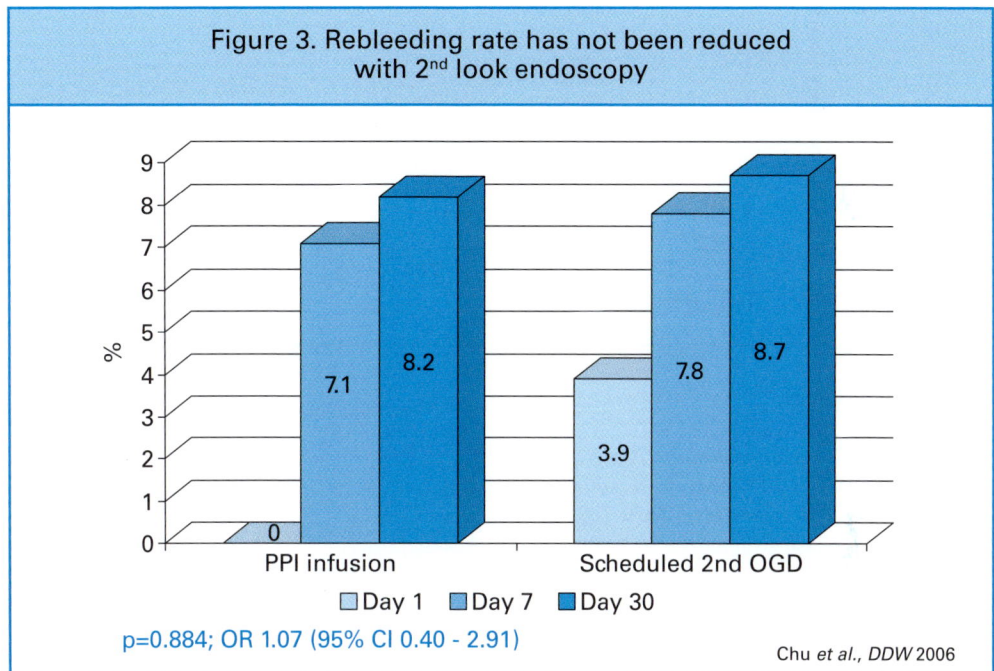

Figure 3. Rebleeding rate has not been reduced with 2nd look endoscopy

p=0.884; OR 1.07 (95% CI 0.40 - 2.91)

Chu et al., DDW 2006

Aspirin has been used in many patients as a primary or secondary prevention of cardiovascular or cerebravascular events. When patients developed ulcer bleeding secondary to aspirin use, there is a dilemma when should this drug be resumed. In a randomized study comparing early resumption of aspirin in patients received high dose PPI and endoscopic hemostasis, mortality was found to be increased with aspirin was withheld until complete ulcer healing. There was, however, a trend, toward increased bleeding rate with early resumption of aspirin. Thus, aspirin is a two-edge sword and discretion of clinicians is required.

Endoscopic therapy do have their limits. When hemostasis cannot be secured, when large underlying vessels (such as gastroduodenal artery) are expected, angiographic hemostasis and surgery should be considered. Detection of these large submucosal or subserosal blood vessels is now possible with the advent of endoscopic ultrasonography.

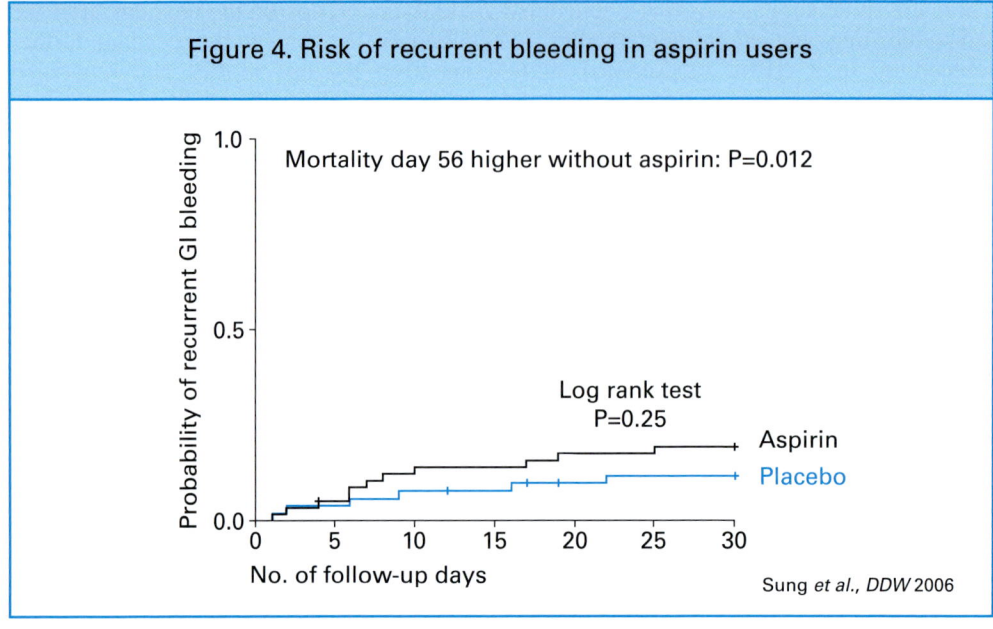

Figure 4. Risk of recurrent bleeding in aspirin users

Selected references

- Calvet X, *et al. Gastroenterology* 2004; 126: 441-50.
- Lanas A, *et al. Gut* 2006 May 10 [Epub ahead of print].
- Sung JJ, *et al. Ann Intern Med* 2003; 139: 237-43.
- Sung JJ, *et al. Gastroenterology* 2006 [abstract DDW 2006].

Role of medical therapy in drug-induced bleeding

Joachim Mössner

University of Leipzig, Germany

About 100 patients per 100,000 inhabitants are hospitalized each year in industrialized Western countries due to significant upper gastrointestinal bleeding [1]. Treatment options include initial resuscitation, prompt endoscopy and, if bleeding cannot be controlled, surgery. Around half of these bleeds are caused by peptic ulcers. The mortality rate in such patients, many of whom are elderly with significant comorbidities [2], is approximately 10% [3].

Non-steroidal anti-inflammatory drugs (NSAIDs) are among the most frequently prescribed medications in Europe and North America. These agents are responsible for several serious gastrointestinal side effects, such as ulcer bleeding. Other drugs, such as polychemotherapy used in treatment of various malignancies, may also but rarely cause gastrointestinal bleeding. However, there are no controlled studies regarding efficiency of medical prophylaxis and treatment in chemotherapy induced gastrointestinal bleeding. In the following we will discuss prophylaxis and medical treatment options of NSAID induced bleeding.

Prostaglandins of the E-type

Prostaglandins of the E-type stimulate, *via* a specific receptor on the parietal cell, the inhibitory G-protein of adenylate cyclase. Thus, they are inhibitors of stimulants, which employ cAMP as second messenger such as histamine-2-receptor antagonists (H$_2$RAs). Besides their slight ability to inhibit acid secretion, prostaglandins stimulate cell regeneration, bicarbonate and mucus secretion.

Prevention of NSAID-induced ulcers

The prostaglandin E1 analogue misoprostol has demonstrated to lower the risk of uncomplicated and complicated NSAID ulcers when given in a dose 4 x 200 µg/day which, however, increases the rate of side effects such as diarrhoea and abdominal pain [4-7]. A small study from Italy reported that misoprostol at 400 – 600 µg/day is significantly more effective than ranitidine (2 x 150 mg/day) in the short-term prevention of naproxen-induced gastric lesions [8]. In another study on patients with NSAID induced upper gastrointestinal pain, misoprostol (4 x 200 µg/day) was significantly more effective than ranitidine (2 x 150 mg/day) in the prevention of NSAID-induced gastric ulcers at 8 weeks. Ranitidine was as effective as misoprostol for the prevention of NSAID-induced duodenal ulcers [9]. In contrast to duodenal ulcers the prevention of NSASD induced gastric ulcers by misoprostol seems to be dose dependent, with misoprostol 800 µg/day being more effective as compared to 400 µg [10]. Since 400 µg/day still offer substantial protection against gastric and duodenal ulcers in patients receiving long-term NSAID therapy, but this dosage causes fewer side effects, misoprostol 2 x 200 µg daily has gained some acceptance. The protective effects of misoprostol against NSAID induced gastrointestinal toxicity prompted the pharmaceutical industry to launch a fixed combination of diclofenac (50 mg) with misoprostol (200 µg). In a double blind, randomized, parallel group study on 361 patients with no significant gastroduodenal lesions, diclofenac/misoprostol (2-3 times/day) was compared with diclofenac/placebo. The fixed combination was associated with less gastroduodenal damage than diclofenac, however, being as effective as diclofenac alone in the treatment of osteoarthritis [11].

A meta-analysis reviewed the effectiveness of various interventions for the prevention of NSAID induced upper gastrointestinal toxicity. Randomized controlled clinical trials using prostaglandin analogues, H_2RAs or proton pump inhibitors (PPIs) were evaluated. Forty randomized controlled trials met the authors' inclusion criteria. All doses of misoprostol significantly reduced the risk of endoscopic ulcers. Misoprostol 800 µg/day was superior to 400 µg/day in prevention of endoscopic gastric ulcers. A dose response relationship was not seen with duodenal ulcers. Misoprostol caused diarrhoea at all doses, although more at 800 µg/day than 400 µg/day. Misoprostol was the only prophylactic agent documented to reduce ulcer complications. Standard doses of H_2RAs were effective at reducing the risk of endoscopic duodenal but not gastric ulcers. Both double dose H_2RAs and PPIs were effective at reducing the risk of endoscopic duodenal and gastric ulcers and were better tolerated than misoprostol. Thus, misoprostol, PPIs, and double dose H_2RAs are effective at preventing chronic NSAID related endoscopic gastric and duodenal ulcers. Lower doses of misoprostol are less effective and are still associated with diarrhoea. Only misoprostol 800 µg/day has been shown to reduce the risk of ulcer perforations, hemorrhages or ulcer obstruction [12].

Proton pump inhibitors

PPIs inhibit the final step of acid secretion, the gastric acid pump. Five proton pump inhibitors are available on the market, omeprazole, esomeprazole, lansoprazole, pantoprazole, and rabeprazole. Tenatoprazole, a further PPI, is not yet available in Europe. All

PPIs are substituted benzimidazoles. They share a similar core structure, 2-pyridyl methyl-sulfinyl benzimidazole, but differ according to substituents on this core. These substitutions are supposed to modify some properties such as 1) chemical stability under acidic and neutral pH, 2) determination with which of the cysteines of the proton pump sulphenamide binding is formed, 3) activation under acidic conditions, 4) pKa values, 5) irreversible inhibition of the pump, 6) half-life, 7) bioavailability, 8) metabolism. Whether these differences in chemical structures translate into differences in clinical efficiency is still a matter of debate.

Peptic ulcers caused by NSAIDs

Omeprazole is more efficient as compared to H_2RAs and misoprostol in treatment of peptic ulcers caused by NSAIDs [13, 14]. There are no meta-analyses comparing various PPIs in various dosages regarding healing rates of NSAID ulcers when NSAID treatment is either stopped or continued.

Prophylaxis of NSAID ulcers

In a prospective, double-blind, multicentre study among 537 patients without *H. pylori* who were both long-term users of NSAIDs and who had a history of documented gastric ulcer the PPI inhibitor lansoprazole (15 or 30 mg/day) was superior to placebo for the prevention of NSAID-induced gastric ulcers but not superior to misoprostol (4 x 200μg/day). The percentages of gastric ulcer-free patients by week 12 were as follows: placebo, 51%; misoprostol, 93%; 15 mg lansoprazole, 80%; and 30 mg lansoprazole, 82%. When the poor compliance and potential adverse effects associated with misoprostol are taken into consideration, PPIs and full-dose misoprostol were clinically equivalent in this study [4]. However, omeprazole has been shown to be more efficient in preventing NSAID ulcers as compared to both ranitidine [14] and a lower dose of misoprostol (2 x 200μg/day) [13]. In a study comparing pantoprazole with misoprostol, patients were randomized to take either pantoprazole (20 mg/day; n = 257) or misoprostol (2 x 200 μg/day; n = 258) for 6 months while continuing NSAID therapy. Remission rates at 3 and 6 months were 93 and 89% for pantoprazole and 79 and 70% for misoprostol. Thus, pantoprazole was superior to the lower dose of misoprostol with regard to prevention of occurrence of ulcers, ten or more erosions/petechiae in the stomach/duodenum, reflux oesophagitis, and severe gastrointestinal symptoms [15].

Furthermore, omeprazole in combination with a non-selective NSAID has been shown to be as efficient in preventing NSAID ulcers as compared to a selective cyclooxygenase II inhibitor such as celecoxib [16]. In ulcers caused by a rather low dose of aspirin, *H. pylori* eradication is as efficient in preventing aspirin ulcers as omeprazole when low dose aspirin is continued [17]. However, omeprazole is more successful in preventing NSAID ulcers as compared to *H. pylori* eradication when a non-selective NSAID such as naproxen is used [17]. Other studies confirmed that NSAID ulcers could be prevented by omeprazole [18] or other PPIs such as lansoprazole [19]. There are no studies comparing various PPIs against one another in treatment and prevention of NSAID ulcers.

Bleeding ulcers

The blood loss of bleeding ulcers can be significant as normal haemostatic mechanisms are impaired in the presence of an acidic environment [20]. Acid suppression may therefore favour haemostasis and reduce rebleeding [20-22]. Despite the fact that in about 80% of cases bleeding stops spontaneously, endoscopic treatment is the standard in acutely bleeding gastric or duodenal ulcers. Endoscopy reduces the rate of rebleeding, need for surgery, and death. However, rebleeding and an overall mortality rate of 10 to 15% remain to be a serious problem. Blood coagulation is hampered by low pH. Thus, elevating the gastric pH should be beneficial. PPIs are highly effective acid-suppressive agents. At present, however, no PPIs are indicated for the prevention of peptic ulcer rebleeding. However, off-label use of intravenous PPIs is very common. According to the results of a study of the Hongkong group [23], at least in Germany common practise is an 80 mg i.v. bolus of either omeprazole, esomeprazole or pantoprazole, followed by continuous infusion of 8 mg/h for 72 hours.

Previous studies have established the benefit of PPI therapy for prevention of peptic ulcer rebleeding [23-25]. The efficacy of PPIs in prevention of rebleeding, surgery, and death was compared with placebo and H_2RAs [26]. The analysis of several randomised, controlled trials [23, 25, 27-29] revealed for PPIs a 50% reduction of the relative odds of rebleeding and 53% reduction for surgery. There was no significant reduction of death. Another meta-analysis demonstrated superiority of PPIs *versus* H_2RAs in preventing persistent or recurrent bleeding from peptic ulcers. However, this beneficial effect seems to be more evident in patients not having endoscopic therapy [30]. Thus, PPIs are superior to H_2RAs. In eight of the nine trials analysed by Zed *et al.*, omeprazole was used primarily intravenously followed by oral medication in some trials. There are no published data comparing other PPIs, which can also be applied intravenously, such as pantoprazole or lansoprazole, with omeprazole or esomeprazole.

Many of these studies, however, were performed in Asia. Thus, their results cannot necessarily be extrapolated to Western populations. For example, the prevalence of *H. pylori* infection is generally higher in Asia than Europe, which has implications for response to acid suppressive therapy [31]. These populations also differ in terms of parietal cell mass [32] and metabolic status. Proportionately more Asian than European patients are slow metabolisers of PPIs because of an increased prevalence of the genetic polymorphism for cytochrome P450 2C19. Thus, a multinational larger scale placebo controlled study is mandatory to clarify whether i.v. PPI therapy is capable to reduce rebleeding and mortality after initial successful endoscopic therapy. The initial success of endoscopic therapy may be a reason of bias regarding the interpretation of some studies of i.v. PPIs. Some previous trials have not distinguished between rebleeding and persistent bleeding (*i.e.* continued bleeding following failed or unattempted endoscopic haemostasis) [33-35]. Furthermore, actively bleeding ulcers, ulcers with nonbleeding visible vessels or clots with underlying vessels are associated with a higher risk of rebleeding as compared to patients with ulcers with clean bases. Thus, patients with these types of ulcers should not be included in a study testing the efficiency of PPIs.

References

1. Longstreth GF. Epidemiology of hospitalization for acute upper gastrointestinal hemorrhage: a population-based study. *Am J Gastroenterol* 1995; 90: 206-10.
2. Higham J, Kang JY, Majeed A. Recent trends in admissions and mortality due to peptic ulcer in England: increasing frequency of hemorrhage among older subjects. *Gut* 2002; 50: 460-4.
3. Rockall TA, Logan RFA, Devlin HB, et al. Incidence and mortality from acute upper gastrointestinal haemorrhage in the United Kingdom. *Br Med J* 1995; 331: 222-6.
4. Graham DY, Agrawal NM, Roth SH. Prevention of NSAID-induced gastric ulcer with misoprostol: multicentre, double-blind, placebo-controlled trial. *Lancet* 1988; 2(8623): 1277-80.
5. Graham DY, White RH, Moreland LW, et al. Duodenal and gastric ulcer prevention with misoprostol in arthritis patients taking NSAIDs. Misoprostol Study Group. *Ann Intern Med* 1993; 119: 257-62.
6. Graham DY, Agrawal NM, Campbell DR, et al. NSAID-Associated Gastric Ulcer Prevention Study Group: Ulcer prevention in long-term users of nonsteroidal anti-inflammatory drugs: results of a double-blind, randomized, multicenter, active- and placebo-controlled study of misoprostol vs lansoprazole. *Arch Intern Med* 2002; 162: 169-75.
7. Silverstein FE, Graham DY, Senior JR, et al. Misoprostol reduces serious gastrointestinal complications in patients with rheumatoid arthritis receiving nonsteroidal anti-inflammatory drugs. A randomized, double-blind, placebo-controlled trial. *Ann Intern Med* 1995; 123: 241-9.
8. Porro GB, Lazzaroni M, Petrillo M: Double-blind, double-dummy endoscopic comparison of the mucosal protective effects of misoprostol *versus* ranitidine on naproxen-induced mucosal injury to the stomach and duodenum in rheumatic patients. *Am J Gastroenterol* 1997; 92: 663-7.
9. Raskin JB, White RH, Jaszewski R, et al. Misoprostol and ranitidine in the prevention of NSAID-induced ulcers: a prospective, double-blind, multicenter study. *Am J Gastroenterol* 1996; 91: 223-7.
10. Raskin JB, White RH, Jackson JE, et al. Misoprostol dosage in the prevention of nonsteroidal anti-inflammatory drug-induced gastric and duodenal ulcers: a comparison of three regimens. *Ann Intern Med* 1995; 123: 344-50.
11. Bolten W, Gomes JA, Stead H, Geis GS. The gastroduodenal safety and efficacy of the fixed combination of diclofenac and misoprostol in the treatment of osteoarthritis. *Br J Rheumatol* 1992; 31: 753-8.
12. Rostom A, Dube C, Wells G, et al. Prevention of NSAID-induced gastroduodenal ulcers. *Cochrane Database Syst Rev* 2002; (4): CD002296.
13. Hawkey CJ, Karrasch JA, Szczepanski L, et al. Omeprazole compared with misoprostol for ulcers associated with nonsteroidal antiinflammatory drugs. Omeprazole *versus* Misoprostol for NSAID-induced Ulcer Management (OMNIUM) Study Group. *New Engl J Med* 1998; 338: 727-34.
14. Yeomans ND, Tulassay Z, Juhasz L, et al. A comparison of omeprazole with ranitidine for ulcers associated with nonsteroidal antiinflammatory drugs. Acid Suppression Trial: Ranitidine versus Omeprazole for NSAID-associated Ulcer Treatment (ASTRONAUT) Study Group. *New Engl J Med* 1998; 338: 719-26.
15. Stupnicki T, Dietrich K, Gonzalez-Carro P, et al. Efficacy and tolerability of pantoprazole compared with misoprostol for the prevention of NSAID-related gastrointestinal lesions and symptoms in rheumatic patients. *Digestion* 2003; 68: 198-208.
16. Chan FK, Hung LC, Suen BY, et al. Celecoxib versus diclofenac and omeprazole in reducing the risk of recurrent ulcer bleeding in patients with arthritis. *N Engl J Med* 2002; 347: 2104-10.
17. Chan FK, Chung SC, Suen BY, et al. Preventing recurrent upper gastrointestinal bleeding in patients with Helicobacter pylori infection who are taking low-dose aspirin or naproxen. *N Engl J Med* 2001; 344: 967-73.
18. Labenz J, Blum AL, Bolten WW, et al. Primary prevention of diclofenac associated ulcers and dyspepsia by omeprazole or triple therapy in Helicobacter pylori positive patients: a randomised, double blind, placebo controlled, clinical trial. *Gut* 2002; 51: 329-35.

19. Lai KC, Lam SK, Chu KM, et al. Lansoprazole reduces ulcer relapse after eradication of Helicobacter pylori in nonsteroidal anti-inflammatory drug users – a randomized trial. *Aliment Pharmacol Ther* 2003; 18: 829-36.
20. Green FW Jr, Kaplan MM, Curtis LE, et al. Effect of acid and pepsin on blood coagulation and platelet aggregation: a possible contributor prolonged gastroduodenal mucosal hemorrhage. *Gastroenterology* 1978; 74: 38-43.
21. Patchett SE, Enright H, Afdhal N, et al. Clot lysis by gastric juice: an *in vitro* study. *Gut* 1989; 30: 1704-7.
22. Li Y, Sha W, Nie Y, et al. Effect of intragastric pH on control of peptic ulcer bleeding. *J Gastroenterol Hepatol* 2000; 15: 148-54.
23. Lau JY, Sung JJ, Lee KK, et al. Effect of intravenous omeprazole on recurrent bleeding after endoscopic treatment of bleeding peptic ulcers. *N Engl J Med* 2000; 343: 310-6.
24. Hasselgren G, Lind T, Lundell L, et al. Continuous intravenous infusion of omeprazole in elderly patients with peptic ulcer bleeding. Results of a placebo-controlled multicenter study. *Scand J Gastroenterol* 1997; 32: 328-33.
25. Lin HJ, Lo WC, Lee FY, et al. A prospective randomized comparative trial showing that omeprazole prevents rebleeding in patients with bleeding peptic ulcer after successful endoscopic therapy. *Arch Intern Med* 1998; 158: 54-8.
26. Zed PJ, Loewen PS, Slavik RS, Marra CA. Meta-analysis of proton pump inhibitors in treatment of bleeding peptic ulcers. *Ann Pharmacother* 2001; 35: 1528-34.
27. Khuroo MS, Yattoo GN, Javid G, et al. A comparison of omeprazole and placebo for bleeding peptic ulcer. *N Engl J Med* 1997; 336: 1054-8.
28. Leontiadis G, McIntyre L, Sharma V, et al. Proton pump inhibitor treatment for acute peptic ulcer bleeding. *Cochrane Database Syst Rev* 2004; (3): CD002094.
29. Bardou M, Toubouti Y, Benhaberou-Brun D, et al. Meta-analysis: proton pump inhibition in high-risk patients with acute peptic ulcer bleeding. *Aliment Pharmacol Ther* 2005; 21: 677-86.
30. Gisbert JP, González L, Calvet X, et al. Proton pump inhibitors versus H2-antagonists: a meta-analysis of their efficacy in treating bleeding peptic ulcer. *Aliment Pharmacol Ther* 2001; 15: 917-26.
31. Van Herwaarden MA, Samsom M, van Nispen CH, et al. The effect of Helicobacter pylori eradication on intragastric pH during dosing with lansoprazole or ranitidine. *Aliment Pharmacol Ther* 1999; 13: 731-40.
32. Lam SK, Hasan M, Sircus W, et al. Comparison of maximal acid output and gastrin response to meals in Chinese and Scottish normal and duodenal ulcer subjects. *Gut* 1980; 21: 324-8.
33. Daneshmend TK, Hawkey CJ, Langman MJ, et al. Omeprazole versus placebo for acute upper gastrointestinal bleeding: randomised double blind controlled trial. *BMJ* 1992; 304: 143-7.
34. Michel P, Duhamel C, Bazin B, et al. Lansoprazole versus ranitidine in the prevention of early recurrences of digestive hemorrhages from gastroduodenal ulcers. Randomized double-blind multicenter study. *Gastroenterol Clin Biol* 1994; 18: 1102-5.
35. Lanas A, Artal A, Blas JM, et al. Effect of parenteral omeprazole and ranitidine on gastric pH and the outcome of bleeding peptic ulcer. *J Clin Gastroenterol* 1995; 21: 103-6.

Is the COX-1, COX-2 hypothesis obsolete?

Richard H. Hunt

McMaster University Health Science Centre, Canada

The understanding of cyclooxygenase (COX)-2 and its role in inflammation and pain provided the potential for a revolution in treatment and was followed by the development of COX-2 selective inhibitors (coxibs), which significantly decreased the incidence of GI complications.

Traditional NSAIDs inhibit both the COX-1 and COX-2 isoforms of cyclo-oxygenase (COX), the enzyme which transforms arachidonic acid into prostaglandins and thromboxanes, which are involved in inflammation, pain and platelet aggregation. COX-1 is expressed in most tissues producing prostanoids that are involved in defence and repair of the GI mucosa, in platelet aggregation and thrombosis, and in some central nervous system pathways regulating pain [1, 2]. COX-2 is expressed constitutively in some tissues including vascular endothelium, kidney and the central nervous system but is induced in most tissues and leucocytes in response to inflammatory stimuli [1].

NSAIDs are amongst the most commonly used medications worldwide for the treatment of pain and inflammation but their use is associated with a high incidence of dyspepsia, GI mucosal injury throughout the GI tract, and serious GI complications including death [3-8]. The main benefits of non-selective NSAIDs (ns-NSAIDs) derives from their anti-inflammatory and analgesic effects, while the main adverse effects are seen in the GI tract and kidneys. Ns-NSAIDs increase the GI complication risk between 3 to 5 fold compared with placebo as demonstrated by several meta-analyses of studies of different design [9]. Ns-NSAIDs associated GI adverse events cause a significant economic burden.

Coxibs have a significantly better GI safety profile than ns-NSAIDs, extensively shown in endoscopy and clinical outcomes studies [7, 10-14]. Compared with traditional NSAIDs, celecoxib is associated with a lower incidence of GI symptoms, including dyspepsia, and is better tolerated thus improving patient compliance [15, 16]. In large outcome studies, symptomatic ulcers and ulcer complications are significantly reduced with first generation coxibs, celecoxib or rofecoxib, compared with ns-NSAID comparators [7, 11, 17]. Although the incidence of adverse events in coxib treated patients increased in relation to the presence of risk factors [18], the differences from ns-NSAIDs was maintained in subgroups of patients with and without risk factors for ulcer complications [19]. Second generation coxibs, such as lumiracoxib and etoricoxib, have greater selectivity for COX-2 and also show improved GI tolerability compared with ns-NSAIDs [12, 20-22]. Meta-analyses further confirm that coxibs are associated with significantly less clinical ulcers and bleeds than ns-NSAIDs [15, 23]. Epidemiological studies also indicate that the introduction of coxibs has been accompanied by a decline in the incidence of GI complications over the last 5-10 years [24, 25], especially in high risk patients [26, 27]. The concomitant use of PPIs and lower doses of ns-NSAIDs also played a role [24]. Coxibs have shown a significantly better safety profile in the lower GI tract when compared with ns-NSAIDs [20, 28-31].

However, recent data have raised concern over the long-term use of coxibs and NSAIDs which have been increasingly associated with a risk of cardiovascular (CV) thrombotic events. Rofecoxib was voluntarily withdrawn from global markets in September 2004 because of an increased risk of myocardial infarction in a prospective randomized placebo-controlled trial for the prevention of recurrent colorectal adenomas [32]. Studies with other first generation coxibs show similar results [33, 34]. Although a numerically higher incidence of adverse CV events was observed when lumiracoxib was compared to naproxen, this was not statistically significant and there were no differences with ibuprofen in the TARGET CV study when high CV risk patients were excluded [35]. The CV risk may be further increased in those who had an indication for, but were not taking, aspirin, rather than in those in whom aspirin was not indicated, or those on long term treatment. Inhibitors of COX also share other potential benefits (*e.g.* cancer preventive effects) and adverse effects (*e.g.* hypertension) [36]. Increasingly, other studies suggest that the increased CV risk observed in some coxib trials is also seen with ns-NSAIDs [37-41]. Several epidemiological studies have also concluded after adjustment for potential confounders, that ns-NSAIDs, coxibs and even acetaminophen increased the risk of serious CV events [38-40, 42]. These new data however challenge the widely held hypothesis that COX-selectivity alone determines the cardiovascular adverse effects of these drugs. The common view is that coxibs increase the risk of cardiovascular thrombotic events by blocking the formation of vasodilatory prostacyclin and leave uninhibited the platelet synthesis of COX-1-mediated thromboxane, which is reversibly affected by ns-NSAIDs [2]. Although coxibs may, by their irreversible covalent binding, strongly impair the synthesis of the antithrombotic prostacyclin and tip the scales of homoeostasis in favour of thrombogenesis and vasoconstriction, there are many other possible factors, including nitric oxide, adiponectin, tissue factor, oxidative stress, etc., which play key and complex roles in this cardiovascular balance [43, 44]. Many of these factors are affected by both coxibs and ns-NSAIDs, and may explain not only a common effect on the cardiovascular system but, also some of the differences observed between these drugs on the cardiovascular risk. Furthermore, the vascular risk associated with long-term NSAID therapy might be mediated in part by an increase in blood pressure, which is affected by both nonselective and selective COX inhibitors [45]. Modest increases or decreases in blood pressure have a rapid impact on cardiovascular and cerebrovascular risk [46].

Aspirin, an irreversible inhibitor of COX-1 and platelet aggregation has specific and unique effects within this class. Aspirin at doses lower than 300 mg/day acts as a selective COX-1 inhibitor and has cardio-vascular protective effects, although it carries dose dependent risks of GI complications [47]. Aspirin is associated with both gastric and duodenal ulcers and upper GI complications occur even with the lowest dose of 75 mg/day [48]. Concomitant ASA and ns-NSAID or coxib treatment carries measurable risk of an adverse upper GI event. Evidence from outcome trials [11, 12, 17], an endoscopy study [49] and epidemiological studies [25, 50] indicate that low-dose aspirin increases further the risk of upper GI bleeding in NSAID users and attenuates the GI benefits of coxibs, but a coxib plus aspirin still provides benefit when compared to co-therapy with an ns-NSAID plus aspirin. Subgroup analyses of GI outcome trials of celecoxib suggest that aspirin with a coxib is associated with a non-significant lower ulcer and ulcer bleeding rate than ns-NSAIDs and aspirin users [11, 17]. Two meta-analyses analyzed tolerability and adverse events in clinical trials of celecoxib in OA and RA patients and both found that celecoxib plus aspirin was associated with a significantly lower endoscopic ulcer rate compared with ns-NSAIDs plus aspirin [15, 51].

The different profiles of ns-NSAIDs and coxibs and recent concerns over both GI and CV adverse effects have caused confusion and complicated the most appropriate management strategies for patients who require effective treatment for pain and inflammation. It has also raised the question of whether the COX-1, COX-2 concepts are obsolete, since there have been a number of new approaches under investigation. These include nitric oxide (NO)-releasing NSAIDs (NO-NSAIDs) or COX inhibiting nitric oxide donating drugs (CINODs) and NO-aspirin and a mixed COX 5- lipoxygenase (LOX) inhibitor [52-55]. The COX inhibiting nitric oxide donor (CINOD) class was designed to provide a multi-pathway mechanism of COX inhibition and nitric oxide donation. NO-releasing aspirin and the COX-inhibiting NO donors, have been considered promising alternatives to ns-NSAIDs with less upper GI toxicity [56, 57]. However, a first study suggests that the renal effects of the NO-NSAID AZD 3582 were similar to those of naproxen and rofecoxib [58]. The first COX 5-LOX inhibitor, licofelone, which inhibits 5-lipoxygenase (5-LOX) COX-1, and COX-2, is being developed based on the hypothesis that inhibition of COX-1/COX-2-mediated arachidonic acid metabolism leads to shunting of arachidonic acid metabolism to leukotrienes (LTs) through the 5-LOX pathway, and LTs are potent gastrotoxic and pro-inflammatory mediators. In theory, a COX 5-LOX inhibitor can inhibit the synthesis of PGs, thromboxanes and LTs and thus reduce production of LTs and PGs, providing similar clinical benefits with a better GI and general tolerability than ns-NSAIDs. GI tolerance has been reported in a study of licofelone in healthy volunteers [59]. However, the efficacy and CV safety of these new medications have not been fully studied, and it is too early to remove the coxibs based on current evidence.

More studies are also needed to understand the mechanisms of NSAIDs gastropathy. Mouse experiments in our lab observed that prostaglandins PGE2 does not inhibit acid secretion in gastric glands from C57BL/6 mice, in contrast to the expected antisecretory effect of PGE2 observed in BALB/c mice. In BALB/c mice the effect of histamine and carbachol was reduced by PGE2, whereas in C57BL/6 mice dose-response curves to these secretagogues were not affected. We subsequently demonstrated that this difference was due to a ~6 fold reduction in the expression of the EP(3) subtype of the PGE receptor, which are not involved in acid secretion in C57BL/6 mice. These host-specific differences in the physiology of acid secretion related to prostaglandins are also likely to be important to the interpretation of the antisecretory role of eicosanoids and the involvement of prostanoids in the etiology of *Helicobacter*-induced inflammation and NSAID-induced gastropathies [60].

Until a new and safer class of NSAIDs is developed to replace the coxibs or ns-NSAIDs, the best therapeutic strategy in the individual patient who needs an NSAID must be based on a careful consideration of the benefits and risks. The benefits derived from the reduction of pain, inflammation and improvement in mobility and quality of life, and those derived from the prevention of CV events with low-dose aspirin, must be balanced against the potential GI and now CV adverse events derived from ns-NSAID or coxib use. From a cost-benefit perspective, prevention strategies should be focused on patients with GI risk factors, which must now to be modified by the presence/absence of CV risk factors [61].

Numerous clinical trials, observational studies and meta-analyses have demonstrated the risk factors which predispose to an NSAID-associated upper GI complication [62, 63]. These include a history of ulcer or ulcer bleeding, increasing age, use of multiple NSAIDs (including low-dose aspirin, high doses of NSAIDs, and concomitant anticoagulant or corticosteroid therapy. There are currently four possible strategies to reduce the risk of GI adverse events associated with ns-NSAID treatment: (1) co-therapy with a gastro-protective drug such as a proton pump inhibitor (PPI) or misoprostol; (2) treatment with a coxib rather than an ns-NSAID; (3) co-therapy with a coxib and a gastro-protective agent in patients at high risk for a GI event; (4) treatment to eradicate *H. pylori* infection in patients with a history of an ulcer with or without complications. Both strategies, the addition of a gastro-protective agent (PPI or misoprostol) to ns-NSAIDs, and the prescription a GI sparing coxib without a gastro-protective agent, are valid for patients without increased CV risk and additional factors. Although the evidence is limited [64], patients with a previous ulcer bleed who need NSAIDs should receive the combination of a coxib plus PPI and *H. pylori* should be tested for and treated if present. Coxib therapy or the combination of a PPI + ns-NSAID are considered to have comparable GI safety profiles in the upper GI tract, whereas coxib treatment seems a better option for the prevention of GI complications from the lower GI tract, although the evidence is still limited. Patients on aspirin that need an NSAID or a coxib may benefit from additional PPI co-therapy. A coxib plus a PPI seems the best therapy for those at the highest GI risk [25, 65, 66], and PPI therapy must be considered for the treatment and prevention of NSAID-induced dyspepsia.

Patients with increased CV risk who require aspirin, other anti-platelet drugs or anticoagulants will also be put at increased risk of developing GI complications if they also take ns-NSAIDs. These patients will benefit from PPI co-therapy regardless of whether they receive an ns-NSAID or a coxib. Although the risk of developing a GI event with the aspirin and coxib (especially low-dose) combination may be lower than the combination of ns-NSAIDs with aspirin, coxibs should be prescribed with caution and all ns-NSAIDs and coxibs should be prescribed at the lowest possible dose and for the shortest time in this setting. In Europe, coxibs are contraindicated in patients with prior CV events and as yet ns-NSAIDs have not been fully reassessed.

References

1. Bolten WW. Scientific rationale for specific inhibition of COX-2. *J Rheumatol* 1998; 51 (Suppl.): 2-7.
2. FitzGerald GA, Patrono C. The coxibs, selective inhibitors of cyclooxygenase-2. *N Engl J Med* 2001; 345 (6): 433-42.
3. Hawkey CJ. Nonsteroidal anti-inflammatory drug gastropathy. *Gastroenterology* 2000; 119: 521-35.
4. Yeomans ND, Lanas A, Talley NJ, Thomson AB, Daneshjoo R, Ericksson B, et al. Prevalence and incidence of gastroduodenal ulcers during treatment with vascular protective doses of aspirin. *Aliment Pharmacol Ther* 2005; 22: 795-801.
5. Brun J, Jones R. Nonsteroidal anti-inflammatory drug-associated dyspepsia: the scale of the problem. *Am J Med* 2001; 110: 12S-13S.
6. Silverstein FE, Graham DY, Senior JR, Davies HW, Struthers BJ, Bittman RM, et al. Misoprostol reduces serious gastrointestinal complications in patients with rheumatoid arthritis receiving nonsteroidal anti-inflammatory drugs. A randomized, double-blind, placebo-controlled trial. *Ann Intern Med* 1995; 123: 241-9.
7. Bombardier C, Laine L, Reicin A, Shapiro D, Burgos-Vargas R, Davis B, et al. Comparison of upper gastrointestinal toxicity of rofecoxib and naproxen in patients with rheumatoid arthritis. VIGOR Study Group. *N Engl J Med* 2000; 343: 1520-8.
8. Tramer MR, Moore RA, Reynolds DJ, McQuay HJ. Quantitative estimation of rare adverse events which follow a biological progression: a new model applied to chronic NSAID use. *Pain* 2000; 85: 169-82.
9. Ofman JJ, et al. Meta-analysis of dyspepsia and nonsteroidal antiinflammatory drugs. *Arthritis Rheum* 2003; 49: 508-18.
10. Silverstein FE, Faich G, Goldstein JL, Simon LS, Pincus T, Whelton A, et al. Gastrointestinal toxicity with celecoxib vs nonsteroidal anti-inflammatory drugs for osteoarthritis and rheumatoid arthritis: the CLASS study: A randomized controlled trial. Celecoxib Long-term Arthritis Safety Study. *JAMA* 2000; 284: 1247-55.
11. Schnitzer TJ, Burmester GR, Mysler E, Hochberg MC, Doherty M, Ehrsam E, et al. Comparison of lumiracoxib with naproxen and ibuprofen in the Therapeutic Arthritis Research and Gastrointestinal Event Trial (TARGET), reduction in ulcer complications: randomised controlled trial. *Lancet* 2004; 364: 665-74.
12. Laine L, Harper S, Simon T, Bath R, Johanson J, Schwartz H et al. A randomized trial comparing the effect of rofecoxib, a cylooxigenase 2-specific inhibitor, with that of ibuprofen on the gastroduodenal mucosa of patients with osteoarthritis. *Gastroenterology* 1999; 117: 776-83.
13. Emery P, Zeidler H, Kvien TK, Guslandi M, Naudin R, Stead H, et al. Celecoxib versus diclofenac in long-term management of rheumatoid arthritis: randomised double-blind comparison. *Lancet* 1999; 354: 2106-11.
14. Moore RA, Derry S, Makinson GT, McQuay HJ. Tolerability and adverse events in clinical trials of celecoxib in osteoarthritis and rheumatoid arthritis: systematic review and meta-analysis of information from company clinical trial reports. *Arthritis Res Ther* 2005; 7: R644-65.
15. Watson DJ, Bolognese JA, Yu C, Krupa D, Curtis S. Use of gastroprotective agents and discontinuations due to dyspepsia with the selective cyclooxygenase-2 inhibitor etoricoxib compared with non-selective NSAIDs. *Curr Med Res Opin* 2004; 20: 1899-908.
16. Singh G, Fort JG, Goldstein JL, Levy RA, Hanrahan PS, Bello AE, et al. Celecoxib versus naproxen and diclofenac in osteoarthritis patients: SUCCESS-I Study. *Am J Med* 2006; 119: 255-66.
17. Skelly MM, Hawkey CJ. Dual COX inhibition and upper gastrointestinal damage. *Curr Pharm Des* 2003; 9: 2191-5.
18. Watson DJ, Yu Q, Bolognese JA, et al. The upper gastrointestinal safety of rofecoxib vs. NSAIDs: an updated combined analysis. *Curr Med Res Opin* 2004; 20: 1539-48.

19. Hunt RH, Harper S, Watson DJ, Yu C, Quan H, Lee M et al. The gastrointestinal safety of the COX-2 selective inhibitor etoricoxib assessed by both endoscopy and analysis of upper gastrointestinal events. *Am J Gastroenterol* 2003; 98: 1725-33.
20. Hawkey CJ, Gitton X, Hoexter G, Richard D, Weinstein WM. Gastrointestinal tolerability of lumiracoxib in patients with osteoarthritis and rheumatoid arthritis. *Clin Gastroenterol Hepatol* 2006; 4: 57-66.
21. Ramey DR, Watson DJ, Yu C, Bolognese JA, Curtis SP, Reicin AS. The incidence of upper gastrointestinal adverse events in clinical trials of etoricoxib vs. non-selective NSAIDs: an updated combined analysis. *Curr Med Res Opin* 2005; 21: 715-22.
22. Goldstein JL, Reduced risk of upper gastrointestinal ulcer complications with celecoxib, a novel COX-2 inhibitor. *Am J Gastroenterol* 2000; 95: 1681-90.
23. Fries JF, Murtagh KN, Bennett M, et al. The rise and decline of nonsteroidal antiinflammatory drug-associated gastropathy in rheumatoid arthritis. *Arthritis Rheum* 2004; 50: 2433-40.
24. Lanas A, Garcia-Rodriguez LA, Arroyo MA, Gomollón F, Zapata E, Bujanda L, et al. Coxibs, NSAIDs, aspirin, PPIs and the risks of upper GI bleeding in common clinical practice. *Gastroenterology* 2005; 128: 629.
25. Mamdani M, Rochon PA, Juurlink DN, Kopp A, Anderson GM, Naglie G, Austin PC, Laupacis A. Observational study of upper gastrointestinal haemorrhage in elderly patients given selective cyclo-oxygenase-2 inhibitors or conventional non-steroidal anti-inflammatory drugs. *BMJ* 2002; 325: 624.
26. Norgard B, Pedersen L, Johnsen SP, Tarone RE, McLaughlin JK, Friis S, Sorensen HT. COX-2-selective inhibitors and the risk of upper gastrointestinal bleeding in high-risk patients with previous gastrointestinal diseases: a population-based case-control study. *Aliment Pharmacol Ther* 2004; 19: 817-25.
27. Goldstein JL, Eisen GM, Lewis B, Gralnek IM, Zlotnick S, Fort JG, Investigators. Video capsule endoscopy to prospectively assess small bowel injury with celecoxib, naproxen plus omeprazole, and placebo. *Clin Gastroenterol Hepatol* 2005; 3: 133-41.
28. Hunt RH, Bowen B, Mortensen ER, Simon TJ, James C, Cagliola A, et al. A Randomized Trial Measuring Fecal Blood Loss after treatment with rofecoxib, Ibuprofen, or placebo in healthy subjects. *Am J Med* 2000; 109: 201-6.
29. Hunt RH, Harper S, Callegari P, Yu C, Quan H, Evans J, James C, Bowen B, Rashid F. Complementary studies of the gastrointestinal safety of the cyclo-oxygenase-2-selective inhibitor etoricoxib. *Aliment Pharmacol Ther* 2003; 17: 201-10.
30. Garner SE, Fidan DD, Frankish R, Maxwell L. Rofecoxib for osteoarthritis. *Cochrane Database Syst Rev* 2005; (1): CD005115.
31. Laine L, Connors LG, Reicin A, Hawkey CJ, Burgos-Vargas R, Schnitzer TJ, et al. Serious lower gastrointestinal clinical events with nonselective NSAID or coxib use. *Gastroenterology* 2003; 124: 288-92.
32. Bresalier RS, Sandler RS, Quan H, Bolognese JA, Oxenius B, Horgan K, Lines C, Riddell R, Morton D, Lanas A, Konstam MA, Baron JA. Adenomatous Polyp Prevention on Vioxx (APPROVe) Trial Investigators. Cardiovascular events associated with rofecoxib in a colorectal adenoma chemoprevention trial. *N Engl J Med* 2005; 352: 1092-102.
33. Solomon SD, McMurray JJ, Pfeffer MA, Wittes J, Fowler R, Finn P, Anderson WF, Zauber A, Hawk E, Bertagnolli M; Adenoma Prevention with Celecoxib (APC) Study Investigators. Cardiovascular risk associated with celecoxib in a clinical trial for colorectal adenoma prevention. *N Engl J Med* 2005; 352: 1071-80.
34. Nussmeier NA, Whelton AA, Brown MT, et al. Complications of the COX-2 inhibitors parecoxib and valdecoxib after cardiac surgery. *N Engl J Med* 2005; 352: 1081-91.
35. Farkouh ME, Kirshner H, Harrington RA, Ruland S, Verheugt FW, Schnitzer TJ,. et al. Comparison of lumiracoxib with naproxen and ibuprofen in the Therapeutic Arthritis Research and Gastrointestinal Event Trial (TARGET), cardiovascular outcomes: randomised controlled trial. *Lancet* 2004; 364: 675-84.

36. Baron JA, Cole BF, Sandler RS, Haile RW, Ahnen D, Bresalier R, *et al.* A randomized trial of aspirin to prevent colorectal adenomas. *N Engl J Med* 2003; 348 (10): 891-9.
37. Konstantinopoulos PA, Lehmann DF. The cardiovascular toxicity of selective and nonselective cyclooxygenase inhibitors: comparisons, contrasts, and aspirin confounding. *J Clin Pharmacol* 2005; 45: 742-50.
38. Hippisley-Cox J, Coupland C. Risk of myocardial infarction in patients taking cyclo-oxygenase-2 inhibitors or conventional non-steroidal anti-inflammatory drugs: population based nested case-control analysis. *Br Med J* 2005; 330: 1366.
39. Ray WA, Stein CM, Hall K, Daugherty JR, Griffin MR. Non-steroidal anti-inflammatory drugs and risk of serious coronary heart disease: an observational cohort study. *Lancet* 2002; 359: 118-23.
40. Chan AT, Manson JE, Albert CM, Chae CU, Rexrode KM, Curhan GC, Rimm EB, Willett WC, Fuchs CS. Nonsteroidal antiinflammatory drugs, acetaminophen, and the risk of cardiovascular events. *Circulation* 2006; 113: 1578-87.
41. Kearney PM, Baigent C, Godwin J, Halls H, Emberson JR, Patrono C.Do selective cyclo-oxygenase-2 inhibitors and traditional non-steroidal anti-inflammatory drugs increase the risk of atherothrombosis? Meta-analysis of randomised trials. *Br Med J* 2006; 332: 1302-8.
42. Helin-Salmivaara A, Virtanen A, Vesalainen R, Gronroos JM, Klaukka T, Idanpaan-Heikkila JE, Huupponen R. NSAID use and the risk of hospitalization for first myocardial infarction in the general population: a nationwide case-control study from Finland. *Eur Heart J* 2006; 27: 1657-63.
43. Crofford LJ, Strand CV, Rushitzka F, Brune K, Farkouh ME, Simon LS.Cardiovascular Effects of Selective COX-2 Inhibition: Is There a Class Effect? The International COX-2 Study Group. *J Rheumatol* 2006; 33: 1403-8.
44. Fosslien E.Cardiovascular complications of non-steroidal anti-inflammatory drugs. *Ann Clin Lab Sci* 2005; 35: 347-85.
45. Pham K, Hirschberg R. Global safety of coxibs and NSAIDs. *Curr Top Med Chem* 2005; 5: 465-73.
46. Staessen JA, Li Y, Thijs L, Wang JG. Blood pressure reduction and cardiovascular prevention: an update including the 2003-2004 secondary prevention trials. *Hypertens Res* 2005; 28: 385-407.
47. Antithrombotic Trialists' Collaboration. Collaborative meta-analysis of randomised trials of antiplatelet therapy for prevention of death, myocardial infarction, and stroke in high risk patients. *Br Med J* 2002 12; 324 (7329): 71-86.
48. Weil J, Colin-Jones D, Langman M, Lawson D, Logan R, Murphy M, *et al.* Prophylactic aspirin and risk of peptic ulcer bleeding. *Br Med J* 1995; 310: 827-30.
49. Laine L, Maller ES, Yu C, Quan H, Simon T. Ulcer formation with low-dose enteric-coated aspirin and the effect of COX-2 selective inhibition: a double-blind trial. *Gastroenterology* 2004; 127: 395-402.
50. Rahme E, Dasgupta K, Toubouti Y, Barkoun AN, Bardou M. GI effect of rofecoxib and celecoxib versus NSAID in patients on low dose aspirin, a population-based retrospective cohort study. *Gastroenterology*, 2004; 126 (4 Suppl. 2), A1 abstract n° 17.
51. Deeks JJ, *et al.* Efficacy, tolerability, and upper gastrointestinal safety of celecoxib for treatment of osteoarthritis and rheumatoid arthritis: systematic review of randomised controlled trials. *Br Med J* 2002; 325: 619.
52. Rainsford KD. The ever-emerging anti-inflammatories. Have there been any real advances? *J Physiol Paris* 2001; 95: 11-9.
53. Zacharowski P, Zacharowski K, Donnellan C, *et al.* The effects and metabolic fate of nitroflurbiprofen in healthy volunteers. *Clin Pharmacol Ther* 2004; 76: 350-8.
54. Hawkey CJ, Jones JI, Atherton CT, *et al.* Gastrointestinal safety of AZD3582, a cyclooxygenase inhibiting nitric oxide donator: proof of concept study in humans. *Gut* 2003; 52: 1537-42.
55. Fiorucci S, Mencarelli A, Meneguzzi A, *et al.* Co-administration of nitric oxide-aspirin (NCX-4016) and aspirin prevents platelet and monocyte activation and protects against gastric damage induced by aspirin in humans. *J Am Coll Cardiol* 2004; 44: 635-41.

56. Lohmander LS, McKeith D, Svensson O, *et al.* A randomised, placebo controlled, comparative trial of the gastrointestinal safety and efficacy of AZD3582 versus naproxen in osteoarthritis. *Ann Rheum Dis* 2005; 64: 449-56.
57. Fiorucci S, Santucci L, Gresele P, *et al.* Gastrointestinal safety of NO-aspirin (NCX-4016) in healthy human volunteers: a proof of concept endoscopic study. *Gastroenterology* 2003; 124: 600-7.
58. Huledal G, Jonzon B, Malmenas M, Hedman A, Andersson LI, Odlind B, Brater DC. Renal effects of the cyclooxygenase-inhibiting nitric oxide donator AZD3582 compared with rofecoxib and naproxen during normal and low sodium intake. *Clin Pharmacol Ther* 2005; 77: 437-50.
59. Bias P, Buchner A, Klesser B, Laufer S. The gastrointestinal tolerability of the LOX/COX inhibitor, licofelone, is similar to placebo and superior to naproxen therapy in healthy volunteers: results from a randomized, controlled trial. *Am J Gastroenterol* 2004; 99 (4): 611-8.
60. Padol I, Hunt RH. Host-specific differences in the physiology of acid secretion related to prostaglandins may play a role in gastric inflammation and injury. *Am J Physiol Gastrointest Liver Physiol* 2005; 288: G1110-7.
61. Scheiman J, Cryer B, Asaka M, Berenbaum F, Bonnet J, Chan FKL, *et al.* Panel Discussion: treatment approaches to control gastrointestinal risk and balance cardiovascular risks and benefits: proposals and recommendations. *Aliment Pharmacol Ther* 2005; Suppl. 1: 26-32.
62. Lanza FL. A guideline for the treatment and prevention of NSAID-induced ulcers. Members of the Ad Hoc Committee on Practice Parameters of the American College of Gastroenterology. *Am J Gastroenterol* 1998; 93: 2037-46.
63. Laine L. Approaches to nonsteroidal anti-inflammatory drug use in the high-risk patient. *Gastroenterology* 2001; 120: 594-606.
64. Chan FKL, Wong VW, Suen BY, Wu JC, Leung WH, Le YT, *et al.* Proton pump inhibitor for the prevention of recurrent ulcer bleeding in patients with arthritis. A double blind, randomized trial. *Gastroenterology* 2006; 130: 133 (A732).
65. Scheiman JM, *et al.* Prevention of Ulcers by Esomeprazole in At-Risk Patients Using Non-Selective NSAIDs and COX-2 Inhibitors. *Am J Gastroenterol* 2006; 101: 701-10.
66. Lanas A, Hunt RH Prevention of anti-inflammatory drug induced GI damage: Benefits and risks of therapeutic strategies. *Ann Med* 2006 (in press).

II

Novel Developments in Gastroenterology. Medical and Surgical Viewpoints

1. Non acid and duodeno-gastro-oesophageal reflux

2. What is really new in the diagnosis and management of intestinal neuropathies and motility disorders?

3. Techniques and indications for minimally invasive procedures

4. New diagnostic tools: ready for clinical application?

Non acid and duodenogastroesophageal reflux
Proofs of concepts and definitions

Daniel Sifrim

Centre for Gastroenterological Research, Catholic University of Leuven, Belgium

Gastroesophageal reflux disease (GERD) arises from an increased exposure and/or sensitivity of the esophageal mucosa to gastric contents. Acid gastroesophageal reflux is essential in the development of GERD and the duration of esophageal acid exposure is a major determinant of the severity of reflux esophagitis [1]. This is the reason why proton pump inhibitors have brought relief to the majority of these patients. Esophageal symptoms and mucosal damage are traditionally related to acid reflux episodes with pH lower than 4. There is a positive correlation between the time elapsed before esophageal pain is experienced and the pH of an esophageal infused solution. The elapsed time to pain sensation increases progressively, eventually leveling off at a pH greater than 4 [2]. Similarly, the degree of mucosal damage can be markedly accelerated if the luminal pH is less than 2 or if active pepsin is present in the refluxate [3].

Esophageal or extraesophageal symptoms of GERD may also be associated with less acidic reflux (pH between 4 and 7) [4-6]. This is the case in both adults and infants after eating, before the gastric contents have become fully acidified and it also applies to reflux in patients undergoing antisecretory therapy.

Although less acidic reflux episodes have been recognized for many years, they were neglected and their real prevalence and clinical relevance remained under investigated. The poor correlation between acid reflux episodes and esophageal or extraesophageal symptoms observed in many patients [7], the high prevalence of non erosive GERD an functional heartburn (not associated with increased esophageal acid exposure) [8] and the persistence of a non-negligible proportion of patients with GERD refractory to adequate PPI therapy [9] has prompted to refocus attention on less acidic reflux episodes as a possible explanation.

Until recently, information about the composition of the refluxate has been limited to data obtained by esophageal pHmetry. However, pH monitoring does not detect gastroesophageal reflux events when little or no acid is present in the refluxate or duodenal alkaline components added to the acid gastric contents. New methodologies have evolved to complement pH monitoring for characterisation of less acidic gastroesophageal reflux. Intraluminal electrical impedance offers the potential to detect and monitor liquid or air movement within the esophageal lumen [10] and Bilitec, a spectrophotometric method, can detect the presence of bilirubin in the refluxate [11]. This review will focuss on the detection of weakly acidic reflux and the current knowledge on its pathophysiology and association with GERD symptoms.

Definitions

Gastroesophageal reflux can be detected by pHmetry alone or, more accurately, by pHmetry combined with intraluminal impedance. Bilirrubin monitoring with Bilitec can distinguish whether or not reflux contains duodeno-pancreatic material.

The pH probe measures acidity at the level of the pH sensor. A pH 4 corresponds to 0.12 meq H^+/litre [12]. The pH measurement gives no indication of the volume of the refluxate, *i.e.* several litres of gastric contents with a pH 2 appear the same to the pH probe as a few millilitres of the same material. Weakly acidic reflux can be detected with pHmetry provided that the pH drop is higher than 1 unit and longer than 4 seconds. However, fluctuations of pH can be due to body movement, respiration or electrode drift. Obviously, if basal esophageal pH is 5, pH-metry will not detect a reflux episode of gastric contents sligthly buffered to pH 4.5.

Using combined pH-manometric parameters, weakly acidic reflux can be detected with the concurrent finding of a pH drop of > 1 unit (between 7 and 4), absent LES pressure and a common cavity phenomenon that ended by primary or secondary peristalsis [13].

In a recent study by Shay and Richter, designed to assess the sensitivity of manometry, pH-metry and impedance for detection of gastroesophageal reflux, manometry could detect 76% of almost 1000 reflux episodes [14].

Intraluminal impedance allows detection of gastroesophageal reflux based on changes in resistance to electrical current flow between two electrodes, when a liquid and/or gas bolus moves between them [10]. The sequence of impedance changes in different segments allows recognition of flow either in aboral (swallow-related) or oral (reflux) directions. Impedance has a sensitivity of at least 90% for detection of all reflux episodes (pH-independent) but does not measure acidity of the intraluminal content.

The use of combined pH monitoring and impedance permits the most accurate detection of reflux episodes. In spite of technical limitations, esophageal bilirubin concentration monitoring (Bilitec) adds information about the chemical nature of material that refluxes into the esophagus.

The term "non-acid" reflux has been used to refer to i) reflux episodes diagnosed by manometry or scintigraphy without pH drops across 4 [15]; ii) duodenogastroesophageal reflux events (DGER) diagnosed with Bilitec monitoring [16]; iii) reflux events diagnosed by impedance monitoring with no change in pH or a drop of pH that does not reach 4 [17] and iv) reflux events diagnosed by impedance monitoring with no change in pH or pH fall of less that 1pH unit [18].

A recent international workshop, that involved experts working in the field of GERD, reviewed and discussed critically the performance of the various tools currently available for detection of gastroesophageal reflux and proposed consensus-based definitions of acid, non-acid and gas reflux, applicable to both adult and paediatric populations [19].

Based on esophageal pH during reflux detected by impedance monitoring three categories of reflux were proposed *(Figures 1, 2 et 3)*.

Acid reflux

Acid reflux is defined as "reflux episodes that decrease esophageal pH across 4, or reflux that occurs when esophageal pH is already below 4".

The occurrence of reflux episodes when the basal esophageal pH is already below 4 represents a special subcategory of acid reflux called "superimposed acid reflux". This is an important phenomenon underlying the delay in esophageal clearance, particularly in patients with hiatal hernia [20, 21].

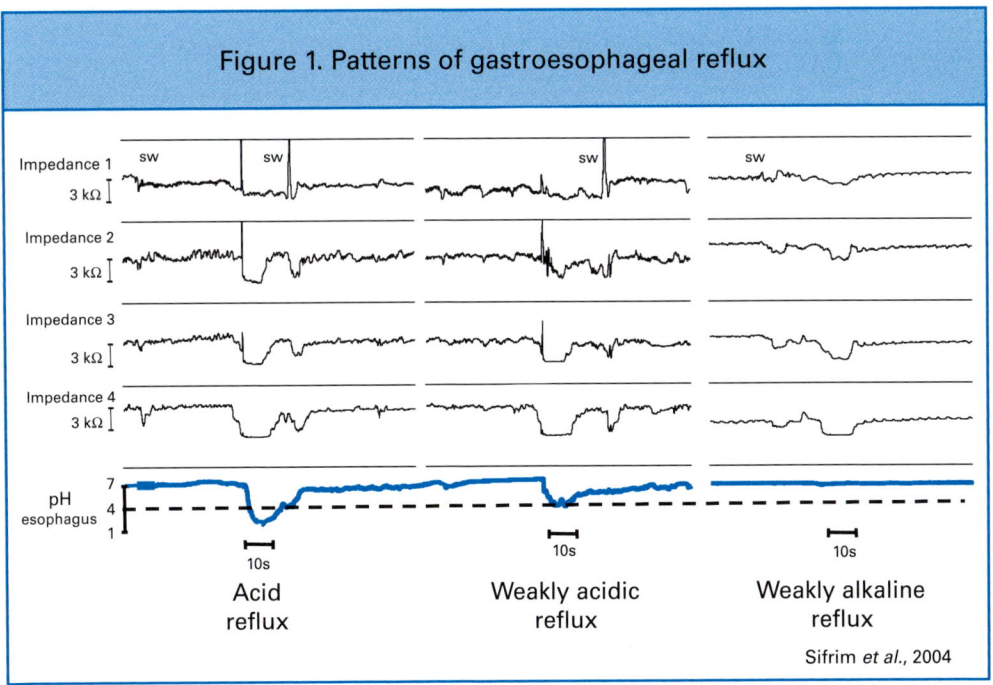

Figure 1. Patterns of gastroesophageal reflux

Sifrim et al., 2004

Figure 2. Gastroesophageal reflux in healthy subjects during 24-Hs ambulatory esophageal impedance - pH monitoring

Total reflux 24hs	Adults (USA) n=60		Adults (Belgium-France) n=72		Premature neonates (Spain) n=22	
	Median	95th percentile	Median	95th percentile	Median	95th percentile
All reflux	30	73	44	75	37	71
Acid reflux	18	55	22	50	16	29
Weakly acidic reflux	9	26	11	33	22	54
Weakly alkaline reflux	0	1	3	15	0	3
Tot ref pH > 4 "non-acid"	9	27	14	48	22	57
	Shay et al., 2004		Zerbib et al., DDW 2004		López et al., DDW 2005	

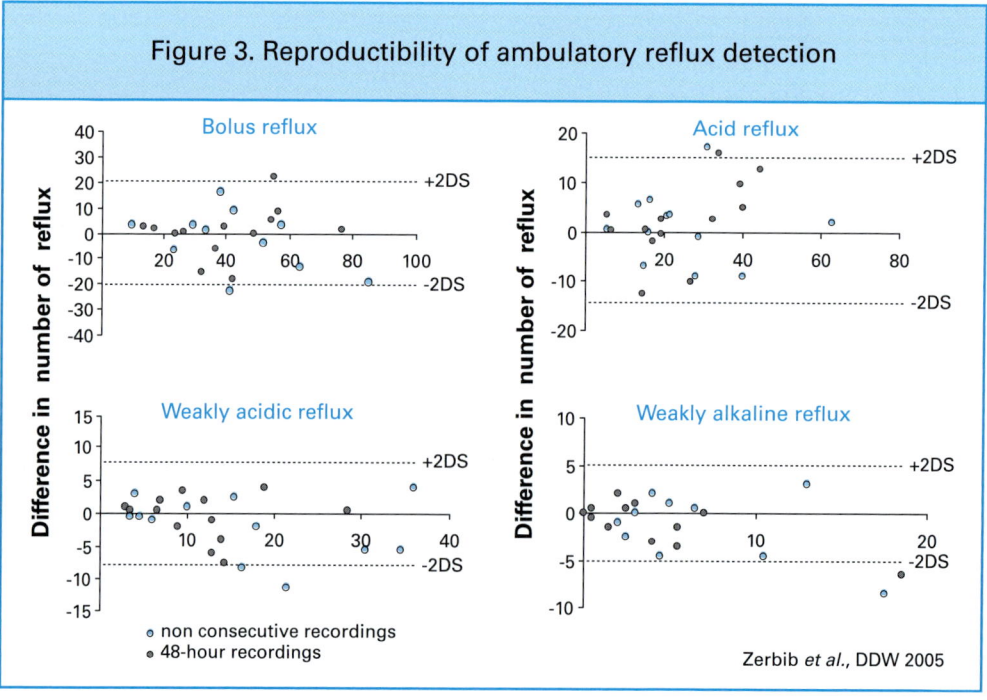

Figure 3. Reproducibility of ambulatory reflux detection

○ non consecutive recordings
● 48-hour recordings

Zerbib et al., DDW 2005

Weakly acidic reflux

All reflux episodes in which the nadir pH lies between 4 and 7 are called "weakly acidic reflux". The upper limit of pH 7 was chosen to define the limit of weakly acidic events, as any fall below pH 7 contains some acid.

Weakly alkaline reflux

The term "weakly alkaline reflux" should be reserved for reflux episodes detected by impedance during which nadir oesophageal pH does not drop below 7.

Previous studies have shown that the term alkaline reflux is a misnomer because esophageal pH changes at/or above 7 do not always correlate with reflux of duodenal contents but rather can be due to swallowed saliva reach in bicarbonate [22, 23].

The term weakly alkaline reflux can now be used because impedance allows the distinction between refluxed or swallowed alkaline material.

Based on the pH of gastric contents that refluxates into the esophagus, the majority of reflux episodes are either acid or weakly acidic. Weakly alkaline reflux is a very exceptional event.

The lack of complete meal homogenisation can explain both, the occurrence of weakly acidic reflux interspersed with episodes of acid reflux and the presence of a local pocket of unbuffered acid in the most proximal stomach. Therefore, weakly acidic reflux is mainly composed by food, gastric mucous secretion and perhaps recently swallowed saliva, pooled in the subcardial region, and poorly mixed with gastric acid.

Does weakly acidic reflux contain duodeno-pancretic material? Aspiration studies suggested that duodeno gastric reflux is a physiological phenomenon occurring mainly postprandially and at night [24]. Therefore, one should expect to detect bile in most postprandial weakly acidic reflux events. However, studies using pH-Bilitec recordings have shown that most DGER events occur in an acid setting, with esophageal luminal pH < 4 [25]. Furthermore, in normal subjects weakly acidic reflux is frequent whereas DGER is rare [26].

It is possible that differences in mixing and distribution of postprandial gastric contents might explain the occurrence of either weakly acidic reflux with little or no bilio-pancreatic secretion or acid DGER containing significant concentration of bile acids. Therefore, a clear distinction should be made between weakly acidic reflux events occurring in the postprandial period of healthy subjects or in patients with GERD under PPI, from acid DGER events, detected with pH-Bilitec, predominantly occurring in patients with moderate and severe GERD [24].

Conclusion

New methodologies have evolved to complement pH monitoring for characterisation of gastroesophageal reflux. Based on acidity and presence of duodeno-pancreatic contents, four types of refluxate can be detected with different prevalence and possible clinical relevance.

– **Acid reflux without duodenal contents** occurs in adults in the fasting and late postprandial periods. Is less common in frequently fed infants. It may have a high proximal extent and is mainly associated with typical GERD symptoms (heartburn and regurgitation) and esophagitis.

– **Acid reflux with duodeno-pancreatic contents** may occur during the postprandial and nocturnal periods with a high proximal extent. It is present in a subgroup of patients with refractory symptoms to PPI therapy and is associated with more severe esophagitis and Barrett's esophagus.

– **Weakly acidic reflux** is mainly present during the postprandial periods in adults and is very common in frequently fed babies. It has a low proximal extent and is not associated with esophagitis, however, it may impair significantly the quality of life in adult patients under PPI with persistent regurgitation or preceding extraesophageal symptoms like chronic cough. The relevance of weakly acidic reflux in endoscopy negative GERD and functional heartburn and for cardiorespiratory events in babies is under investigation.

– **Weakly alkaline reflux** is very rare and it has a similar symptom association profile than weakly acidic reflux.

References

1. Ghillebert G., Demeyere AM, Janssens J, Vantrappen G. How well can quantitative 24-hour intraesophageal pH monitoring distinguish various degrees of reflux disease? *Dig Dis Sci* 1995; 40: 1317-24.
2. Smith JL, Opekun AR, Larkai E, Graham DY. Sensitivity of the esophageal mucosa to pH in gastroesophageal reflux disease. *Gastroenterology* 1989; 96: 683-9.
3. Richter J. Do we know the cause of reflux disease? *Eur J Gastroenterol Hepatol* 1999; 11 (Suppl. 1): S3-9.
4. Dent J, Holloway RH, Toouli J, Dodds WJ. Mechanisms of lower oesophageal sphincter incompetence in patients with symptomatic gastrooesophageal reflux. *Gut* 1988; 29: 1020-8.
5. Breumelhof R, Nadorp JH, Akkermans LM, Smout AJ. Analysis of 24-hour esophageal pressure and pH data in unselected patients with noncardiac chest pain. *Gastroenterology* 1990; 99: 1257-64.
6. Mattioli S, Pilotti V, Felice V, Lazzari A, Zannoli R, Bacchi ML, et al. Ambulatory 24-hr pH monitoring of esophagus, fundus, and antrum. A new technique for simultaneous study of gastroesophageal and duodenogastric reflux. *Dig Dis Sci* 1990; 35: 929-38.
7. Colas-Atger E, Bonaz B, Papillon E, Gueddah N, Rolachon A, Bost R, et al. Relationship between acid reflux episodes and gastroesophageal reflux symptoms is very inconstant. *Dig Dis Sci* 2002; 47: 645-51.

8. Galmiche JP, des Varannes SB. Endoscopy-negative reflux disease. *Curr Gastroenterol Rep* 2001; 3: 206-14.
9. Kahrilas PJ. Refractory heartburn. *Gastroenterology* 2003; 124: 1941-5.
10. Silny J. Intraluminal multiple electrical impedance procedure for measurement of gastrointestinal motility. *J Gastrointest Mot* 1991; 3: 151-62.
11. Bechi P, Pucciani F, Baldini F, Cosi F, Falciai R, Mazzanti R, et al. Long-term ambulatory enterogastric reflux monitoring. Validation of a new fiberoptic technique. *Dig Dis Sci* 1993; 38: 1297-306.
12. Shay SS, Bomeli S, Richter J. Multichannel intraluminal impedance accurately detects fasting, recumbent reflux events and their clearing. *Am J Physiol Gastrointest Liver Physiol* 2002; 283: G376-83.
13. Wyman JB, Dent J, Holloway RH. Changes in oesophageal pH associated with gastro-oesophageal reflux. Are traditional criteria sensitive for detection of reflux? *Scand J Gastroenterol* 1993; 28: 827-32.
14. Shay S, Richter J. Direct comparison of impedance, common cavity, and pH probe in detecting daytime GER's and their characteristics. *Gastroenterology* 2003; 124: A534 (abstract).
15. Washington N, Moss HA, Washington C, Greaves JL, Steele RJ, Wilson CG. Non-invasive detection of gastro-oesophageal reflux using an ambulatory system. *Gut* 1993; 34: 1482-6.
16. Katz PO. Review article: the role of non-acid reflux in gastro-oesophageal reflux disease. *Aliment Pharmacol Ther* 2000; 14: 1539-51.
17. Vela MF, Camacho-Lobato L, Srinivasan R, Tutuian R, Katz PO, Castell DO. Simultaneous intraesophageal impedance and pH measurement of acid and nonacid gastroesophageal reflux: effect of omeprazole. *Gastroenterology* 2001; 120: 1599-606.
18. Sifrim D, Silny J, Holloway RH, Janssens JJ. Patterns of gas and liquid reflux during transient lower oesophageal sphincter relaxation: a study using intraluminal electrical impedance. *Gut* 1999; 44: 47-54.
19. Sifrim D, Castell D, Dent J, Kahrilas P. Gastroesophageal reflux monitoring: review and consensus report on detection and definitions of acid, non-acid and gas reflux. *Gut* 2004; 53: 1024-31.
20. Mittal RK, Lange RC, McCallum RW. Identification and mechanism of delayed esophageal acid clearance in subjects with hiatus hernia. *Gastroenterology* 1987; 92: 130-5.
21. Kahrilas PJ. Anatomy and physiology of the gastroesophageal junction. *Gastroenterol Clin North Am* 1997; 26: 467-86.
22. Singh S, Bradley LA, Richter JE. Determinants of oesophageal 'alkaline' pH environment in controls and patients with gastro-oesophageal reflux disease. *Gut* 1993; 34: 309-16.
23. Penagini R, Yuen H, Misiewicz JJ, Bianchi PA. Alkaline intra-oesophageal pH and gastro-oesophageal reflux in patients with peptic oesophagitis. *Scand J Gastroenterol* 1988; 23: 675-8.
24. Schindlbeck NE, Heinrich C, Stellaard F, Paumgartner G, Muller-Lissner SA. Healthy controls have as much bile reflux as gastric ulcer patients. *Gut* 1987; 28: 1577-83.
25. Vaezi M, Richter J. Role of acid and duodenogastroesophageal reflux in gastroesophageal reflux disease. *Gastroenterology* 1996; 111: 1192-9.
26. Tack J, Bisschops R, Koek G, Sifrim D, Lerut T, Janssens J. Dietary restrictions during ambulatory monitoring of duodenogastroesophageal reflux. *Dig Dis Sci* 2003; 48: 1213-20.

Novel Developments in Gastroenterology.
P. Malfertheiner, L. Lundell, G. Tytgat, eds. John Libbey Eurotext, Paris © 2006, pp. 53-62.

The role of bile and pepsin in the pathophysiology and treatment of gastro-esophageal reflux disease

Jan Tack

Department of Gastroenterology, University Hospital Gasthuisberg, Leuven, Belgium

Summary

Gastro-eesophageal reflux disease (GERD) is a multifaceted and multifactorial disorder which results from the reflux of gastric contents into the oesophagus. Animal studies suggest that synergism between acid and pepsin and conjugated bile acids have the greatest damaging potential for esophageal mucosa, although unconjugated bile acids may be caustic at more neutral pH. Human studies are compatible with a synergistic action between acid and duodenogastric reflux in inducing lesions. During prolonged monitoring studies, typical GORD symptoms are more related to acid reflux events than to non-acid reflux events. However, symptoms that persist during acid suppressive therapy are often related to non-acid reflux events. The therapeutic options for the non-acid component of the refluxate, including acid suppression, prokinetics, baclofen, surgery, and mucosal protective agents like alginates, are discussed.

Key points

A. Animal studies and human studies suggest that a synergism between acid, pepsin and bile is involved in the pathogenesis of GERD-related lesions.
B. In the absence of acid suppressive therapy, typical GORD symptoms are mainly related to acid reflux events.
C. Typical GERD symptoms that persist during acid suppressive therapy are more likely to be related to non-acid reflux events.
D. Only few studies addressed the treatment of the non-acid component in GERD. Modalities include prokinetics, baclofen, surgery, and mucosal protective agents like alginates.

Gastro-esophageal reflux disease (GERD) is defined as the presence of symptoms or lesions that can be attributed to the reflux of gastric contents into the oesophagus [1]. The most typical clinical symptoms are heartburn and regurgitation, whereas peptic esophagitis and Barrett's oesophagus are the typical lesions, but GORD can manifest itself through a multitude of less typical presentations. When effects of refluxed gastric contents extend beyond the oesophagus itself, this is referred to as extra-oesophageal reflux. Extra-oesophageal manifestations of GORD include a variety of pulmonary and ear, nose and throat (ENT) symptoms and disorders, which have been summarized in the literature [2].

Although incompletely understood, it is clear that the pathophysiology of gastro-esophageal reflux disease is multifactorial. The pressure of the lower esophageal sphincter, the motility of the esophageal body and the stomach, the composition of the reflux material, and the sensitivity or resistance of the esophageal mucosa to the reflux material, are important factors involved in the pathogenesis of GERD-related symptoms and lesions [3].

The refluxate is not only composed of gastric acid and pepsin, but may also contain food and regurgitated duodenal contents [4, 5]. In adults, reflux of duodenal contents into the stomach is a physiological event, especially in the postprandial period and during the night [6, 7]. Hence, is not unusual for the contents of material that refluxes into the esophagus to contain duodenal contents, and this is referred to as duodenogastroesophageal reflux (DGER).

Measurement of pepsin bile reflux

No device is available that allows measuring pepsin exposure of the esophagus over prolonged periods of time. Hence, investigations of the role of pepsin have been limited to indirect evidence, like assessment of pH ranges at which pepsin is active [8, 9], short-term aspiration studies [10-13], and studies that demonstrate the presence of pepsin in extra-esophageal locations [14-16].

The methods to study DGER have recently been reviewed [5]. The role of DGER has initially been evaluated by means of endoscopy with biopsies [17, 18], scintigraphy [19], aspiration studies [10-13] and esophageal pH monitoring. It has been assumed that alkaline pH on pH monitoring represented "bile reflux", [20], but it is now well established that "alkaline reflux" is not equivalent with DGER [20, 21]. Stationary aspiration studies were able to demonstrate the presence of bile in esophageal aspirates from patients with esophagitis [10, 11]. More recently, a method for ambulatory refluxate aspiration was developed. This confirmed that reflux into the esophagus of both bile and pancreatic enzymes occur frequently in patients with reflux disease [13].

The Bilitec 2000® (Synectics Medical, Sweden) device is a fiberoptic spectrophotometric probe developed to quantify DGER in an ambulatory way. Bilirubin, present in bile, has a characteristic absorption band at 450 mm. *In vitro* validation studies confirmed a good correlation between the total bilirubin concentration of aspirated samples and the fiberoptic reading of bilirubin concentration [13]. Moreover, a good correlation was found between concentrations of bilirubin and pancreatic enzymes in aspirated refluxate. Based on these observations, bilirubin seems to be an accurate tracer for DGER monitoring in patients who have normal serum bilirubin levels.

The intraluminal esophageal impedance technique detects gastroesophageal reflux events based on changes in resistance to electrical current flow between pairs of electrodes [22]. The method allows detection of several types of reflux events, regardless of whether they are liquid (drop in impedance) or gas (increase in impedance) or mixed [23, 24]. It is often assumed that DGER and non-acid reflux detected by impedance monitoring represent the same event. However, combined pH, bilitec, with or without impedance, studies have shown that the DGER component usually accompanies acid reflex events, and that the non-acid component on impedance monitoring studies is not equivalent to bile reflux [25].

Role of pepsin and bile in esophageal lesions

In vitro studies

The contribution of different factors present in the refluxate on esophageal integrity was studied in several *in vitro* animal models. Most studies, summarized by Vaezi *et al.* in 1996, have indicated that the esophageal mucosa is relatively resistant to acid exposure alone, whereas the addition of pepsin or bile salts (conjugated at acidic pH, unconjugated at more neutral pH) induce lesions at more physiological levels of acid exposure [26-31]. More recent studies have confirmed this concept, have investigated underlying mechanisms and expanded it to supra-esophageal lesions.

In the cat esophagus *in vivo*, Pursnani *et al.* found no additive damaging effect of pepsin above the effect of acid perfusion [32]. On the other hand, recent studies on rabbit esophageal cells *in vitro* confirmed that pepsin and acid produced more lesions than acid alone [33-35]. This process seemed to involve superoxide anion generation and could be partially inhibited by the free radical scavenger superoxide dismutase [36]. Pre-exposure to acidified saline induced a protective adaptation, diminishing damage during subsequent acid and pepsin perfusion [34]. A study on the dog larynx, investigating mechanisms of extra-esophageal injury in GERD, concluded that pepsin and combinations of pepsin with conjugated bile acids in acidic environments were the principal caustic factors [37]. In a porcine larynx model, exposure to acid was shown to induce squamous epithelial proteins Sep70 and Sep53, whereas acid with pepsin depleted these putatively protective proteins [38].

Taken together, these observations demonstrate synergism between acid, pepsin and bile acids in triggering a number of molecular events that lead to esophageal damage. Proteolytic enzymes like pepsin or trypsin cause direct tissue damage and release of intracellular mediators. The mechanism through which bile acids may contribute to lesions are less clear. Through damage to lipid membranes, they may also induce release of intracellular mediators. In the murine colon, bile acids induce mast cell degranulation and release of histamine and prostaglandins [39]. It is unclear whether similar events contribute to the effects of bile acids in the esophagus.

Barrett's esophagus with it's risk for adenocarcinoma is the most severe complication of GERD. In rats, surgery that induces duodeno-esophageal reflux is associated with the development of columnar lined epithelium and adenocarcinoma [40]. Mediators that are potentially involved in the malignant degeneration of Barrett's esophagus, like COX-2, are induced in cultured rat esophageal cells by exposure to bile acids [41]. In *in vitro* studies of the human esophagus, synergistic damaging effects of HCl with pepsin and bile acids have been reported [42, 43]. In human Barrett's epithelium and esophageal adenocarcinoma *in vitro*, the proto-ongogene C-myc is up-reglated, and expression is increased by exposure to bile acids [44].

Clinical studies

In man, the respective role of acid and DGER in inducing esophageal lesions is incompletely elucidated. In partial gastrectomy patients, excessive DGER is demonstrable in the majority, but esophagitis seems confined to a subset with excessive gastro-esophageal acid reflux [45]. Several studies using combined pH and DGER monitoring in non-operated GERD patients suggest increasing amounts of acid reflux and of DGER with increasing severity of esophageal lesions, especially in patients with Barrett's esophagus and complicated Barrett's esophagus [46-51]. The results of these studies are supportive of a synergistic activity of acid and bile reflux in inducing esophageal lesions.

A multivariate analysis revealed that long-lasting reflux episodes, as well as the presence of a hiatal hernia and a defective esophageal sphincter, were independent risk factors associated with the presence of Barrett's esophagus [52]. In a recent study, analyzing demographic characteristics and parameters derived from 24 hour ambulatory esophageal pH and Bilitec® monitoring and esophageal manometry, we found that presence of esophagitis was associated with duodeno-gastro-esophageal reflux exposure, and that the severity of esophagitis was associated with esophageal acid exposure [53]. Male sex, acid exposure and duodeno-gastro-esophageal reflux exposure are all independent risk factors for the presence of Barrett's esophagus. These data confirm the role of duodeno-gastro-esophageal reflux as an independent risk factor for reflux-associated lesions, and they also demonstrate the multifactorial nature of the pathophysiology of reflux-related lesions.

A number of observations suggest that DGER in the absence of acid reflux may also be sufficient to induce lesions. It has been reported that total gastrectomy patients may still develop severe esophagitis [54]. In critically ill patients, receiving stress ulcer prophylaxis with ranitidine, the presence of esophagitis was significantly correlated with the presence of pathological DGER [55]. These data support the role of DGER in the genesis of esophageal lesions, even in the absence of an acid component *(Figure 1)*.

Recent studies have also explored the contribution of acid and pepsin to supra-esophageal lesions in man. In patients with presumed laryngopharyngeal reflux (LPR), decreased laryngeal expression of carbonic anhydrase and E-cadherin was reported [56]. In LPR patients, the presence of pepsin in laryngeal epithelial cells, probably through receptor-mediated uptake, was associated with decreased expression of squamous epithelial proteins Sep70 and Sep53 [38]. These observations are suggestive of pepsin-induced loss of cellular defenses in the laryngeal epithelium.

The role of pepsin and bile in esophageal symptoms

The relationship between acid reflux episodes and symptoms has been extensively studied. Acid perfusion studies established that HCl at pH 2 or lower is able to induce heartburn in all patients studied, suggesting a major role for acid in inducing heartburn [57]. Recently, it was demonstrated that esophageal perfusion of bile acids is also able to induce heartburn [58].

During ambulatory pH monitoring studies, less than half of the reported heartburn episodes in GERD patients are associated with acid reflux [59, 60]. Two studies using combined acid and DGER reflux monitoring found that most symptom episodes were associated with acid reflux alone or mixed reflux, while less than 10% were associated with bile reflux alone [59, 60]. These observations indicate that symptom episodes in patients with presumed gastro-esophageal reflux disease are much more often related to acid reflux than to bile reflux. Duodeno-gastro-esophageal reflux therefore does not seem to be important in producing typical esophageal symptoms. The role of DGER in atypical symptoms has not been studied to a large extent.

When symptomatic patients are studied while on acid suppressive therapy, a high proportion of symptomatic episodes is related to non-acid reflux, as measured with esophageal impedance monitoring [61]. Similarly, bile reflux monitoring on PPI revealed a higher proportion of symptom episodes related to DGER as compared to acid reflux events [62] *(Figure 1)*.

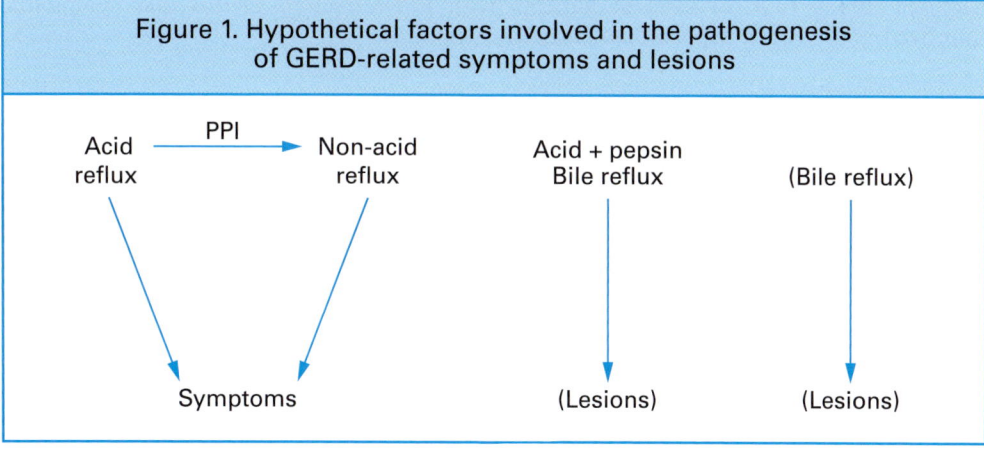

In the absence of acid suppressive therapy, typical GORD symptoms are mainly related to acid reflux events. Typical GERD symptoms that persist during acid suppressive therapy are more likely to be related to non-acid reflux events. Animal studies and human studies suggest that a synergism between acid, pepsin and bile is involved in the pathogenesis of GERD-related lesions. Under specific, more rare circumstances, non-acid reflux alone seems to underlie the pathogenesis of esophageal lesions.

Therapeutic implications

Acid suppression

Proton pump inhibitors are the cornerstone of GERD treatment. Several studies have shown that treatment with proton pump inhibitors dramatically decreases both acid and DGER as measured by a Bilitec probe [46, 63-65]. It has been suggested that the effects of PPIs on DGER is indirect, mediated by the ability of proton pump inhibitors to decrease both gastric acidity and volume. However, the available literature suggests that PPIs are less efficacious to normalise DGER, compared to their effect on acid reflux [46, 63-65]. In GERD patients with symptoms that persist during PPI therapy, particularly high prevalences of persisting pathological DGER have been reported [62].

Prokinetics and surgery

The therapeutic approach to patients with persisting DGER has not been well established. It seems logical that prokinetics may improve DGER, but this has only been demonstrated in partial gastrectomy patients using high doses of cisapride [66], which is no longer available due to cardiac adverse events. Anti-reflux surgery was shown to adequately reverse DGER [64], but not all patients are suitable candidates for surgical therapy.

Baclofen

Transient lower esophageal sphincter relaxations (TLESRs) are the main pathophysiological mechanism underlying gastro-esophageal reflux events [67, 68]. The GABA B agonist baclofen was shown to decrease the number of TLESRs in health and in GERD, thereby potentially decreasing all reflux events [69, 70]. In one uncontrolled study adding baclofen 20 mg t.i.d. to PPIs in patients with PPI-refractory DGER and symptoms, improved both DGER exposure and GERD symptoms [71].

Mucosal protection

In view of the involvement of toxic radicals and cellular membrane degenration in the pathogenesis of GERD lesions, there is a role for locally acting mucosal protective therapy. In a rat model of mixed reflux, a novel anti-oxidant decreased the severity of esophagitis and the expression of cellular markers of esophageal damage [72]. Human studies with this or other anti-oxydants are lacking.

Alginates are biopolymers derived from algae, which have seen applications as thickeners, stabilisers, gel-forming and film-forming agents. *In vitro* studies suggest a number of properties of alginates that offer a potential for protection against bile or pepsin. Alginates bind to esophageal mucosa, interact with mucin [73, 74], inhibit diffusion and activity of pepsin [75, 76], and have immune stimulating properties as well [77]. Studies investigating the effects of alginates in GERD patients on a molecular level seem warranted.

References

1. Kahrilas PJ, Quigley FM. Clinical esophageal pH recording: a technical review for practice guideline development. *Gastroenterology* 1996; 110: 1982-96.
2. Poelmans J, Tack J. Extraoesophageal manifestations of gastro-oesophageal reflux. *Gut* 2005; 54: 1492-9.
3. Tack J. Recent developments in the pathophysiology and therapy of gastroesophageal reflux disease and nonerosive reflux disease. *Curr Opin Gastroenterol* 2005; 21: 454-60.
4. Vaezi MF, Singh S, Richter JE. Role of acid and duodenogastric reflux in esophageal injury: a review of animal and human studies. *Gastroenterology* 1995; 108: 1897-907.
5. Tack J. Review article: role of pepsin and bile in gastro-esophageal reflux disease. *Aliment Pharmacol Ther* 2005; 22 (Suppl. 1): 48-54.
6. Mearin F, Azpiroz F, Malagelada JR, Zinsmeister AR. Antroduodenal resitence to flow in the control of duodenogastric bile reflux during fasting. *Gastroenterology* 1987; 93: 1026-33.
7. Koek G, Vos R, Sifrim D, Cuomo R, Janssens J, Tack J. Mechanisms underlying duodeno-gastric reflux in man. *Neurogastroenterol Motil* 2005; 17: 191-9.
8. Bremner RM, Crookes PF, DeMeester TR, Peters JH, Stein HJ. Concentration of refluxed acid and esophageal mucosal injury. *Am J Surg* 1992; 164: 522-6.
9. Dent J. Roles of gastric acid and pH in the pathogenesis of gastro-oesophageal reflux disease. *Scand J Gastroenterol* 1994; 201 (Suppl.): 55-61.
10. Gotley DC, Morgan AP, Ball D, Owens RW, Cooper MJ. Bile acid concentrations in the refluxate of patients with reflux oesophagitis. *Br J Surg* 1988; 75: 587-90.
11. Johnsson F, Joelsson B, Floren CH, *et al*. Bile salts in the esophagus of patients with esophagitis. *Scand J Gastroenterol* 1988; 23: 712-6.
12. Gotley DC, Morgan AP, Ball D, Owen RW, Cooper MJ. Composition of gastro-oesophageal refluxate. *Gut* 1991; 32: 1093-9.
13. Stipa F, Stein HJ, Feussner H, Kraemer S, Siewert JR. Assessment of non-acidic esophageal reflux: comparison between long-term reflux aspiration test and fiberoptic bilirubin monitoring. *Dis Esophagus* 1997; 10: 24-8.
14. Tasker A. Dettmar PW, Panetti M, Koufman JA, Birchall JP, Pearson JP. Reflux of gastric juice and glue ear in children. *Lancet* 2002; 359: 493.
15. Tasker A. Dettmar PW, Panetti M, Koufman JA, Birchall JP, Pearson JP. Is gastric reflux a cause of otitis media with effusion in children? *Laryngoscope* 2002; 112: 1930-4.
16. Metheny NA, Chang YH, Ye JS, Edwards SJ, Defer J, Dahms TE, Stewart BJ, Stone KS, Clouse RE. Pepsin as a marker for pulmonary aspiration. *Am J Crit Care* 2002; 11: 150-4.
17. Nasrallah SM, Johnston GS, Gadacz TR, *et al*. The significance of gastric bile reflux at endoscopy. *J Clin Gastroenterol* 1987; 9: 514-7.
18. Stein HJ, Smyrck TC, DeMeester TR, *et al*. Clinical value of endoscopy and histology in the diagnosis of duodenogastric reflux disease. *Surgery* 1992; 112: 796-804.
19. Drane WE, Karvelis K, Johnson DA, *et al*. Scintigrafic evaluation of duodenogastric reflux. Problems, pitfalls and technical review. *Clin Nucl Med* 1987; 12: 377-84.
20. Singh S, Bradley LA, Richter JE. Determinants of esophageal alkaline pH environment in controls and patients with gastroesophageal reflux disease. *Gut* 1993; 34: 309-16.
21. Devault KR, Georgson S, Castell DO: Salivary stimulation mimics esophageal exposure to refluxed duodenal contents. *Am J Gastroenterol* 1993; 88: 1040-3.
22. Fass J, Silny J, Braun J, Heindrichs U, Dreuz B, Schumpelick V, Rau G. Measuring esophageal motility with a new intraluminal impedance device. First clinical results in reflux patients. *Scand J Gastroenterol* 1994; 29: 693-720.
23. Sifrim D, Holloway R, Silny J, Tack J, Lerut A, Janssens J. Composition of the postprandial refluxate in patients with gastroesophageal reflux disease. *Am J Gastroenterol* 2001; 96: 647-55.

24. Sifrim D, Holloway R, Silny J, Xin Z, Tack J, Lerut A, Janssens J. Acid, nonacid, and gas reflux in patients with gastroesophageal reflux disease during ambulatory 24-hr pH-Impedance recordings. *Gastroenterology* 2001; 120: 1588-98.
25. Sifrim D, Castell D, Kent J, Kahrilas PJ. Gastro-oesophageal reflux monitoring: review and consensus report on detection and definitions of acid, non-acid and gas reflux. *Gut* 2004; 53: 1024-31.
26. Vaezi MF, Singh S, Richter JE. Role of acid and duodenogastric reflux in esophageal mucosal injury: a review of animal and human studies. *Gastroenterology* 1995; 108: 1897-907.
27. Goldberg HI, Dodds WJ, Gee S, Montgomery C, Zboralske FF. Role of acid and pepsin in acute experimental esophagitis. *Gastroenterology* 1969; 56: 223-30.
28. Harmon JW, Johnson LF, Maydonovitch CL. Effects of acid and bile salts on the rabbit esophageal mucosa. *Dig Dis Sci* 1981; 26: 65-72.
29. Lillemoe KD, Johnson LF, Harmon JW. Role of the components of the gastroduodenal contents in experimental acid esophagitis. *Surgery* 1982; 92: 276-84.
30. Salo JA, Kivilaakso E. Contribution of trypsin and cholate to the pathogenesis of experimental alkaline reflux esophagitis. *Scand J Gastroenterol* 1984; 19: 875-81.
31. Johnson LF, Harmon JW. Experimental esophagitis in a rabbit model. Clinical relevance. *J Clin Gastroenterol* 1986; 8 (Suppl. 1): 26-44.
32. Pursnani KG, Mohiuddin MA, Geisinger KR, Weinbaum G, Katzka DA, Castell DO. Experimental study of acid burden and acute oesophagitis. *Br J Surg* 1998; 85: 677-80.
33. Lanas A, Royo Y, Ortego J, Molina M, Sainz R. Experimental esophagitis induced by acid and pepsin in rabbits mimicking human reflux esophagitis. *Gastroenterology*. 1999; 116: 97-107.
34. Lanas AI, Blas JM, Ortego J, Soria J, Sainz R. Adaptation of esophageal mucosa to acid- and pepsin-induced damage: role of nitric oxide and epidermal growth factor. *Dig Dis Sci* 1997; 42: 1003-12.
35. Tobey NA, Hosseini SS, Caymaz-Bor C, Wyatt HR, Orlando GS, Orlando RC. The role of pepsin in acid injury to esophageal epithelium. *Am J Gastroenterol* 2001; 96: 3062-70.
36. Naya MJ, Pereboom D, Ortego J, Alda JO, Lanas A. Superoxide anions produced by inflammatory cells play an important part in the pathogenesis of acid and pepsin induced oesophagitis in rabbits. *Gut* 1997; 40: 175-81.
37. Adhami T, Goldblum JL, Richter JE, Vaezi MF. The role of gastric and duodenal agents in laryngeal injury: an experimental canine model. *Am J Gastroenterol* 2004; 99: 2098-106.
38. Johnston N, Dettmar PW, Lively MO, Postma GN, Belafsky PC, Birchall M, Koufman JA. Effect of pepsin on laryngeal stress protein (Sep70, Sep53, and Hsp70) response: role in laryngopharyngeal reflux disease. *Ann Otol Rhinol Laryngol* 2006; 115: 47-58.
39. Gelbmann CM, Schteingart CD, Thompson SM, Hofmann AF, Barrett KE. Mast cells and histamine contribute to bile acid-stimulated secretion in the mouse colon. *J Clin Invest* 1995; 95: 2831-9.
40. Miwa K, Sahara H, Segawa M, Kinami S, Sato T, Miyazaki I, Hattori T. Reflux of duodenal or gastro-duodenal contents induces esophageal carcinoma in rats. *Int J Cancer* 1996; 67: 269-74.
41. Zhang F, Altorki NK, Wu YC, Soslow RA, Subbbaramaiah K, Dannenberg AJ. Duodenal reflux induces cyclooxygenase-2 in the esophageal mucosa of rats: evidence for involvement of bile acids. *Gastroenterology* 2001; 121: 1391-9.
42. Hopwood D, Bateson MC, Milne G, Bouchier IA. Effects of bile acids and hydrogen ion on the fine structure of oesophageal epithelium. *Gut* 1981; 22: 306-11.
43. Gotley DC, Flaks B, Cooper MJ. Bile acids do not modify the effects of pepsin on the fine structure of human oesophagal epithelium. *Auts NW J Surg* 1992; 62: 579-75.
44. Tselepis C, Morris CD, Wakelin D, Hardy R, Perry I, Luong QT, Harper E, Harrison R, Atwood SE, Jankowski JA. Upregulatio nof the oncogene c-myc in Barrett's adenocarcinoma: induction of c-myc by acified bile acid in vitro. *Gut* 2003; 52: 174-80.
45. Sears RJ, Champion GL, Richter JE. Characteristics of distal partial gastrectomy patients with oesophageal symptoms of duodeno-gastric reflux. *Am J Gastroenterol* 1995; 90: 211-5.

46. Champion G, Richter JE, Vaezi MF, Singh S, Alexander R. Duodeno-gastro-esophageal reflux: relationship to pH and importance in Barrett's esophagus. *Gastroenterology* 1994; 107: 747-54.
47. Caldwell MT, Lawlor P, Byrne PJ, Walsh TN, Hennessy TP. Ambulatory oesophageal bile reflux monitoring in Barrett's esophagus. *Br J Surg* 1995; 82: 657-60.
48. Vaezi MF, Richter JE. Synergism of acid and duodenogastroesophageal reflux in complicated Barrett's esophagus. *Surgery* 1995; 117: 699-704.
49. Kauer WK, Peters JH, DeMeester TR, Ireland AP, Bremner CG, Hagen JA. Mixed reflux of gastric and duodenal juices is more harmful to the esophagus than gastric juice alone. The need for surgical therapy re-emphasized. *Ann Surg* 1995; 222: 525-31.
50. Cuomo R, Koek G, Sifrim D, Janssens J, Tack J. Analysis of ambulatory duodenogastroesophageal reflux monitoring. *Dig Dis Sci* 2000; 45: 2463-9.
51. Tack J, Bisschops R, Koek G, Sifrim D, Lerut T, Janssens J. Dietary restrictions during ambulatory monitoring of duodenogastroesophageal reflux. *Dig Dis Sci* 2003; 48: 1213-30.
52. Campos GM, DeMeester SR, Peters JH, Oberg S, Crookes PF, Hagen JA, Bremner CG, Sillin LF, Mason RJ, DeMeester TR. Predictive factors of Barrett esophagus: multivariate analysis of 502 patients with gastroesophageal reflux disease. *Arch Surg* 2001; 136: 1267-73.
53. Koek GH, Degreef A, Sifrim D, Janssens J, Tack J. A multivariate analysis of pathophysiological factors in reflux esophagitis and Barrett's esophagus: acid reflux, bile reflux or both? Submitted for publication.
54. Orlando RC, Bozymski EM. Heartburn in pernicious anemia – a consequence of bile reflux. *N Engl J Med* 1973; 289: 522-3.
55. Wilmer A, Tack J, Frans E, Dits H, Vanderschueren S, Gevers A, Bobbaers H. Duodenogastroesophageal reflux and esophageal mucosal injury in mechanically ventilated patients. *Gastroenterology* 1999; 116: 1239-9.
56. Johnston N, Bulmer D, Gill GA, Panetti M, Ross PE, Pearson JP, Pignatelli M, Axford SE, Dettmar PW, Koufman JA. Cell biology of laryngeal epithelial defenses in health and disease: further studies. *Ann Otol Rhinol Laryngol* 2003; 112: 481-91.
57. Smith JL, Opekun AR, Larkai E, Graham DY. Sensitivity of the eospahgeal mucosa to pH in gastroesophageal reflux disease. *Gastroenterology* 1989; 96: 683-9.
58. Siddiqui A, Rodriguez-Stanley S, Zubaidi S, Miner PB. Esophageal visceral sensitivity to bile salts in patients with functional heartburn and in healthy control subjects. *Dig Dis Si* 2005; 50: 81-5.
59. Marshall RE, Anggiansah A, Owen WA, Owen WJ. The relationship between acid and bile reflux and symptoms in gastro-esophageal reflux disease. *Gut* 1997; 40: 182-7.
60. Koek GH, Tack J, Sifrim D, Lerut T, Janssans J. The role of acid and duodenal gastroesophageal reflux in symptomatic GERD. *Am J Gastoenterol* 2001; 96: 2033-40.
61. Vela M, Camacho-Lobato L, Srinivasan R, Tutuian R, Katz PO, Castell DO. Simultaneous intraesophageal impedance and pH measurement of acid and nonacid gastroesophageal reflux: Effect of Omeprazole. *Gastroenterology* 2001; 120: 1599-606.
62. Tack J, Koek G, Demedts I, Sifrim D, Janssens J. Gastro-esophageal reflux disease poorly responsive to single dose proton pump inhibitors in patients without Barrett's esophagus: acid reflux, bile reflux or both? *Am J Gastroenterol* 2004; 99: 981-9.
63. Marshall RE, Anggiansah A, Manifold DK, Owen WA, Owen WJ. Effect of omeprazole 20 mg twice daily on duodenogastric and gastro-osophageal bile reflux in barrett's esophagus. *Gut* 1998; 43 : 603-6.
64. Stein HJ, Kauer WK, Feussner H, and Siewert JR. Bile reflux in benign and malignant Barrett's esophagus: effect of medical acid suppression and Nissen fundoplication. *J Gastrointest Surg* 1998; 2: 333-41.
65. Menges M, Muller M, Zeitz M. Increased acid and bile reflux in Barrett's esophagus compared to reflux esophagitis, and effect of proton pump inhibitor therapy. *Am J Gastroenterol* 2001; 96: 331-7.

66. Vaezi MF, Sears R, Richter JE. Placebo-controlled trial of cisapride in postgastrectomy patients with duodenogastroesophageal reflux. *Dig Dis Sci* 1996; 41: 754-63.
67. Penagini R, Schoeman MN, Dent J, Tippett MD, Holloway R. Motor events underlying gastro-esophageal reflux in ambulant patients with reflux esophagitis. *Neurogastroenterol Mot* 1996; 8: 131-41.
68. Schoeman MN, Tippett MD, Akkermans LMA, Dent J, Holloway RH. Mechanisms of gastroesophageal reflux in ambulant healthy human subjects. *Gastroenterology* 1995; 108: 83-91.
69. Lidums I, Lehmann A, Cheklin H, Dent J, Holloway RH. Control of transient lower esophageal sphincter relaxations and reflux by the GABA (B) agonist baclofen in normal subjects. *Gastroenterology* 2000; 118: 7-13.
70. Zhang Q, Lehmann A, Rigda R, Dent J, Holloway RH. Control of transient lower esophageal sphincter relaxations and reflux by the GABA (B) agonist baclofen in patients with gastro-oesophageal reflux disease. *Gut* 2002, 05: 19-24.
71. Koek GH, Sifrim D, Lerut T, Janssens J, Tack J. The effect of the GABAb agonist baclofen in patients with symptoms and duodenogastro-esophageal reflux refractory to proton pump inhibitors. *Gut* 2003; 10: 1397-402.
72. Oh TY, Lee JS, Ahn BO, Cho H, Kim WB, Kim YB, Surh YJ, Cho SW, Lee KM, Hahm KB. Oxidative stress is more important than acid in the pathogenesis of reflux oesophagitis in rats. *Gut* 2001; 49: 364-71.
73. Batchelor H, Craig D, Dettmar PW, Jolliffe I, Hampson F. Investigation into the rheological synergy between salivary mucins and alginate. 19th Pharmaceutical Technology Conference; 2000; 1: 39-43.
74. Richardson JC, Dettmar PW, Hampson FC, Melia CD. Oesophageal bioadhesion of sodium alginate suspensions: particle swelling and mucosal retention. *Eur J Pharm Sci* 2004; 23: 49-56.
75. Tang M, Dettmar P, Batchelor H. Bioadhesive oesophageal bandages: protection against acid and pepsin injury. *Int J Pharm* 2005; 292: 169-77.
76. Strugala V, Kennington EJ, Campbell RJ, Skjak-Braek G, Dettmar PW. Inhibition of pepsin activity by alginates in vitro and the effect of epimerization. *Int J Pharm* 2005; 304: 40-50.
77. Flo TH, Ryan L, Kilaas L, Skjak-Braek G, Ingalls RR, Sundan A, Golenbock DT, Espevik T. Involvement of CD14 and beta2-integrins in activating cells with soluble and particulate lipopolysaccharides and mannuronic acid polymers. *Infect Immun* 2000; 68: 6770-6.

Impedance pH monitoring

Radu Tutuian

Division of Gastroenterology and Hepatology, University Hospital Zurich, Zurich, Switzerland

Proton pump inhibitors (PPI) had a major impact on the management of gastroesophageal reflux disease (GERD). Within 8 weeks of treatment PPIs heal erosive esophageal lesions in 90% of patients underscoring the importance of gastric acid in the pathogenesis of esophageal mucosal damage. On the other hand GERD symptoms persist in 30-35% of patients treated with daily doses of PPIs, often despite the healing of esophagitis. In this situation it becomes important to evaluate whether persistent symptoms on PPI therapy are due to ongoing acid or non-acid reflux or not related to reflux. The concept of "non-acid" reflux has been introduced to describe reflux episodes not readily detected by conventional pH monitoring. Over the years radiography, scintigraphy, bilirubin monitoring and impedance monitoring have been used to overcome the limitations of pH monitoring in detecting gastroesophageal reflux. This presentation will focus primarily on using multichannel intraluminal impedance (MII) combined with pH (MII-pH) to monitor gastroesophageal reflux.

Principles of impedance-pH monitoring

Intraluminal impedance monitoring exploits differences in electrical conductivity of the esophageal wall and intraluminal content to detect the presence of liquids or gas within the esophageal lumen [1]. Placing two metal rings separated by an isolator in the esophageal lumen and applying alternating electrical current between the two rings, one will measure within this circuit the baseline impedance (*i.e.* resistance to alternating current) of the esophageal mucosa. The presence of liquid between these two rings (*i.e.* impedance measuring segment) will improve the electrical conductivity leading to a decrease in impedance while the presence of gas/air between in the impedance measuring segment will produce a rise in impedance as air has poor electrical conductivity *(Figure 1)*. Mounting several impedance measuring segments on the same catheter (*i.e.* multichannel intraluminal impedance) one can measure not only the presence of intraluminal content at

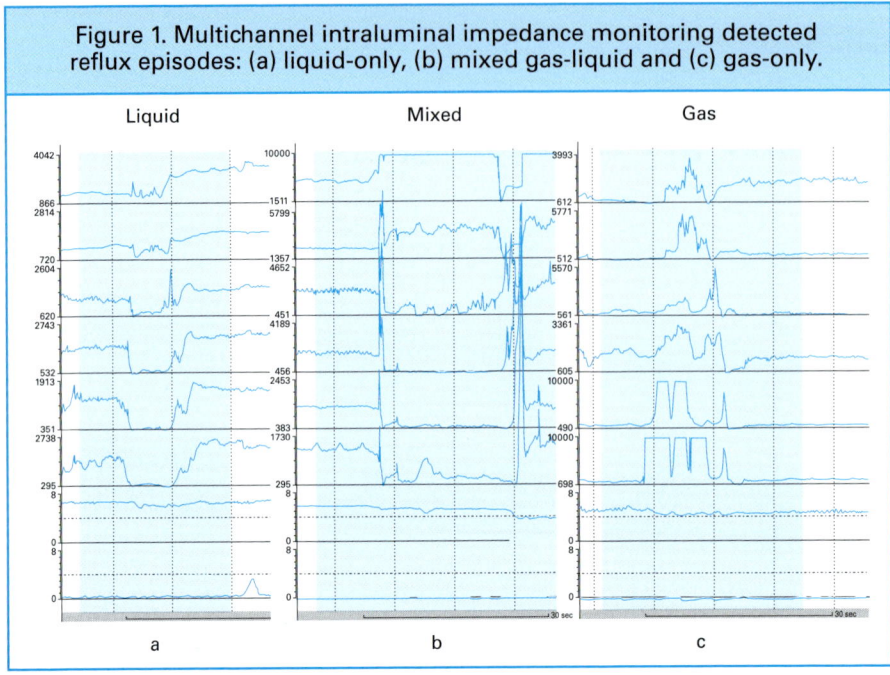

Figure 1. Multichannel intraluminal impedance monitoring detected reflux episodes: (a) liquid-only, (b) mixed gas-liquid and (c) gas-only.

multiple levels but also determine the direction of bolus movement within the esophagus. Drops in impedance advancing over time from proximal to distal indicate an antegrade bolus movement as seen during liquid swallowing, while drops in impedance advancing over time from distal to proximal indicate a retrograde bolus movement as seen during liquid reflux episodes. Adding a pH electrode to the system allows monitoring the H^+ activity of the intraluminal content and classifies reflux episodes as acid or non-acid.

The high sensitivity of detecting the presence of liquid within the esophageal lumen is, on the other hand a drawback of this technology when it comes to measuring volumes. Since 1ml and 10ml of liquid are producing the same changes, impedance cannot be accurately be used to determine the volume [2].

Characteristics of reflux episodes using impedance-pH monitoring

Combined impedance-pH monitoring brings not only a shift in the reflux testing paradigm but also the need for new definitions. In combined MII-pH monitoring reflux MII identifies reflux episodes and provides information on the physical properties of reflux episodes such as liquid, gas or mixed composition and height of the reflux episodes. The pH sensor provides data which allows classifying reflux episodes into acid or non-acid based on pre-established criteria. Currently there are two trends in the literature when it comes to the classification of reflux episodes with a pH above 4. One school of thought tries combining the gastrointestinal and chemical definition of acid and alkaline proposing to define acid reflux episodes MII-detected reflux episodes with a drop in pH from above to below 4, weakly acidic reflux episodes MII-detected reflux episodes with a nadir pH between 4-7 and weakly alkaline reflux episodes MII-detected reflux episodes with a pH above 7 [3]. The second school of thought proposes a more pragmatic approach using the same definition for acid reflux and defines non-acid reflux MII-detected reflux episodes with a nadir pH above 4 since "weakly alkaline" reflux episodes are very rare [4]. For the reader it is therefore important to recognize that the terms "non-acid" and "weakly acidic" can be used interchangeably.

Clinical application of impedance-pH monitoring

An important step in establishing the clinical value of impedance-pH monitoring was establishing normal values. Currently there are three multicenter studies reporting similar normal values in US-Belgian, French-Belgian and Italian cohorts of healthy volunteers not taking acid suppressive medications (*i.e.* "off therapy"). Based on these studies up to 73 MII-detected reflux episodes are considered normal and the main benefit of adding MII to conventional pH monitoring is in the post-prandial period when food is buffering the intragastric acidity and less than half of reflux episodes have a pH below 4.0 (*i.e.* acid reflux episodes). So far normal values "on therapy" have been established in a group of 20 healthy volunteers while taking twice daily 40mg of esomeprazole and these preliminary data indicate that the upper limit of normal "on therapy" should be 48 MII-detected reflux episodes.

More important than characterizing the amount of normal or abnormal number of reflux episodes is evaluating the relationship of symptoms with reflux episodes. Bredenoord *et al.* monitored 32 patients with typical GERD symptoms off therapy and found that only 11% of reflux episodes are symptomatic [5]. The authors noted that compared with asymptomatic episodes, symptomatic episodes were associated with a larger pH drop, lower nadir pH and higher proximal extent and that symptomatic reflux episodes had a longer volume and acid clearance time.

Early studies on acid suppressive therapy by Vela *et al.* found that non-acid reflux can also be associated with heartburn and regurgitation [6]. More recently, in a multicenter study including 168 patients on PPI bid, Mainie *et al.* noted that "on therapy" 48% of symptomatic patients referred to tertiary care centers had a positive symptom index (SI) for acid (11%) or non-acid (37%) reflux and 52% had a negative SI [7]. A positive SI was more often noted in patients with typical symptoms (52%) than in patients with atypical symptoms (22%).

The clinical relevance of this association is underscored by the observation of Mainie *et al.* in 19 patients with symptomatic non-acid reflux which underwent laparoscopic fundoplication [8]. During the post-operative follow-up (average 14 months) after fundoplication 16/18 (89%) patients with a positive SI for non-acid reflux on PPI therapy were asymptomatic and not taking acid suppressive medications. Although these observations do not include a control group these preliminary data indicate that symptomatic non-acid is of clinical relevance and laparoscopic fundoplication can be a treatment option for patients with documented association between symptoms and non-acid reflux.

Conclusions

Impedance-pH monitoring represents a novel clinical tool to monitor gastroesophageal reflux. In the opinion of several investigators it is the ideal tool to monitor patients with persistent symptom on acid suppressive therapy as it allows evaluating whether persistent symptoms on PPI therapy are associated with reflux (acid and non-acid) or not associated with reflux *(Figure 2)*. The ability to document this association opens a new door for discussions on the optimal treatment of patients with symptomatic acid and non-acid reflux on PPI therapy.

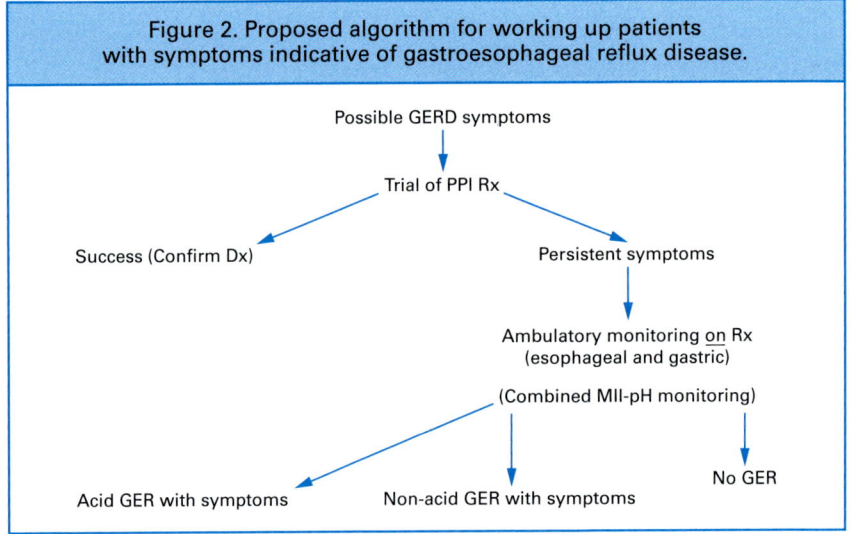

Figure 2. Proposed algorithm for working up patients with symptoms indicative of gastroesophageal reflux disease.

References

1. Silny J. Intraluminal multiple electric impedance procedure for measurement of gastrointestinal motility. *J Gastrointest Motil* 1991; 3: 151-62.
2. Srinivasan R, Vela MF, Katz PO, Tutuian R, Castell JA, Castell DO. Esophageal function testing using multichannel intraluminal impedance. *Am J Physiol* 2001; 280: G457-62.
3. Sifrim D, Castell D, Dent J, Kahrilas PJ. Gastro-oesophageal reflux monitoring: review and consensus report on detection and definitions of acid, non-acid, and gas reflux. *Gut* 2004; 53: 1024-31.
4. Tutuian R, Vela MF, Shay SS, Castell DO. Multichannel Intraluminal Impedance (MII) in esophageal function testing and gastroesophageal reflux monitoring. *J Clin Gastroenterol* 2003; 37: 206-15.
5. Bredenoord AJ, Weusten BL, Curvers WL, Timmer R, Smout AJ. Determinants of perception of heartburn and regurgitation. *Gut* 2006; 55: 313-8.
6. Vela M, Camacho-Lobato L, Srinivasan R, Tutuian R, Katz PO, Castell DO. Simultaneous intraesophageal impedance and pH measurement of acid and nonacid gastroesophageal reflux: effect of omeprazole. *Gastroenterology* 2001; 120: 1599-606.
7. Mainie I, Tutuian R, Shay S, Vela M, Zhang X, Sifrim D, Castell DO. Acid and non-acid reflux in patients with persistent symptoms despite acid suppressive therapy. A multicenter study using combined ambulatory impedance-pH monitoring. *Gut* 2006; in press.
8. Mainie I, Tutuian R, Agrawal A, Adams D, Castell DO. Combined multichannel intraluminal impedance-pH monitoring identifies patients with persistent reflux symptoms on acid suppressive therapy who benefit from a laparoscopic Nissen fundoplication. *Br J Surg* 2006; in press.

Non-acid and duodeno-gastro-oesophageal reflux: therapeutic options

Jean Paul Galmiche

Institut des Maladies de l'Appareil Digestif, Hôtel-Dieu, Nantes, France

Gastro-oesophageal reflux disease (GORD) is a very common disorder in which the reflux of gastric (or gastro-duodenal) contents causes troublesome symptoms and/or lesions of the oesophageal mucosa. The harmful effects of acid on the oesophageal mucosa have been established for decades by experimental and clinical studies. However, despite the progress made with PPIs, up to 40% of patients with reflux symptoms and/or lesions of oesophagitis are either not completely satisfied with their acid-suppressive therapy or may be resistant to PPIs. Thus, besides the significant role of acid in GORD pathogenesis, other components of the reflux material can also exert a deleterious effect upon the oesophageal mucosa.

The non-acid components of the reflux material include biliary acids and enzymes such as trypsin, normally present into the duodenum, which can reflux into the stomach and then reach the oesophagus leading to the so-called duodeno-gastro-oesophageal reflux (DGOR). These molecules *(Figure 1)* can act either alone or synergistically with acid. This has important therapeutic consequences as acid suppression may also contribute to a reduction of the non-acid aggression. Moreover, a reduction of the volume of fluids present in the stomach may also reduce the trigger for transient lower oesophageal sphincter relaxations (TLOSRs), the main mechanism of both acid and biliary reflux episodes.

Several studies have actually shown that PPIs are able to reduce not only oesophageal acid exposure, but also bilirubin exposure (a marker of biliary reflux detected by Bilitec technology). However, the terms "non-acid reflux" and "biliary reflux" are not equivalent. With the development of oesophageal impedance monitoring systems which can detect virtually all reflux episodes, it has been rapidly established that not all acid reflux episodes reach the pH threshold of 4, a threshold arbitrarily set for the classical definition of "acid reflux" in former pH studies. In fact, weakly acidic reflux episodes (*i.e.* reflux events shown by change in impedance levels associated with a pH drop that does fall below pH 4) can be responsible for reflux symptoms; these include both typical and atypical manifestations such as regurgitation and cough, for example. Similarly, although far less frequently, symptoms can be triggered by weakly alkaline reflux episodes (reflux episodes during which nadir oesophageal pH does not drop below 6.5).

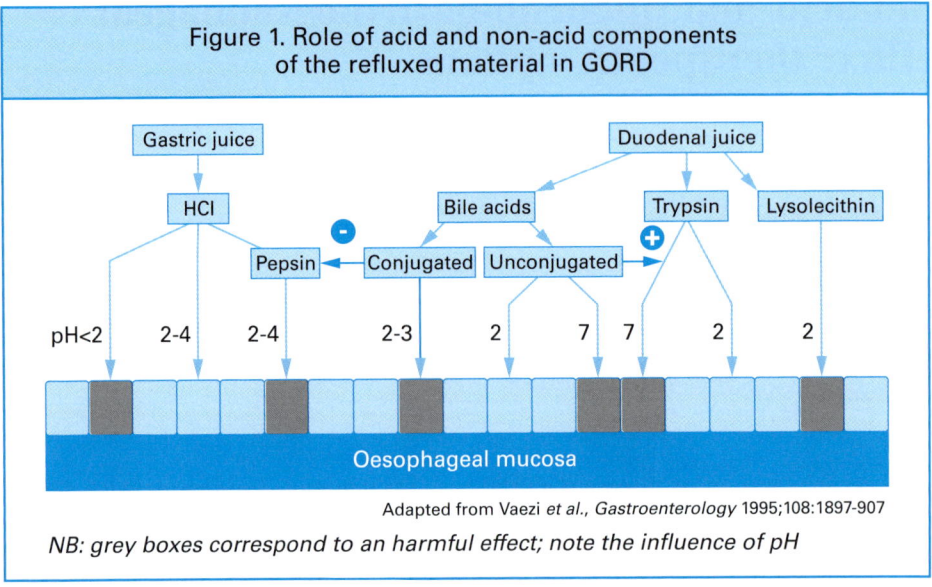

Figure 1. Role of acid and non-acid components of the refluxed material in GORD

Adapted from Vaezi *et al.*, *Gastroenterology* 1995;108:1897-907

NB: grey boxes correspond to an harmful effect; note the influence of pH

These new definitions are very useful for research purposes but so far impedance-pH monitoring is not widely available or, in reality, fully validated for clinical application. In fact, very few pharmacological or therapeutic trials have been conducted in reflux patients well-characterised at baseline with respect to DGOR (Bilitec) and/or non-acid reflux (pH-impedance). However, preliminary studies which have usually arisen from the same groups can provide some guidance for a strategy to be followed in the practical setting.

In practice, a diagnosis of non-acid reflux is usually suspected in patients who are poor responders to PPIs. The management of patients with suspected non-acid (or DGOR) reflux should be a step-by-step approach. After checking for compliance and adequate prescribing of a PPI, it is always important to reconsider the diagnosis of GORD itself. Indeed, a substantial proportion of PPI-non responders do not have acid reflux. This can ideally be shown by pH-monitoring and careful symptom analysis after discontinuation of acid suppression when there is a temporal relationship between symptoms and reflux episodes. Adding impedance to pH monitoring slightly increases the diagnostic yield, however relatively few patients are in fact resistant to PPIs because of an inadequate control of oesophageal acid exposure. In contrast, pH-impedance monitoring is most useful when performed in a patient on-therapy as shown in *Figure 2*. In patients with weakly acidic reflux related symptoms, it seems logical to try a therapeutic regimen using a high dose PPI (*e.g.* double or triple dose PPI daily) or a combination of a PPI and H2-blocker (although pharmacological tolerance frequently occurs rapidly with the latter compound). In the future, long-acting PPIs with prolonged plasma half-lives such as tenatoprazole (or its isomer S-tenatoprazole sodium) may help to optimise the control of acid secretion, especially during the night.

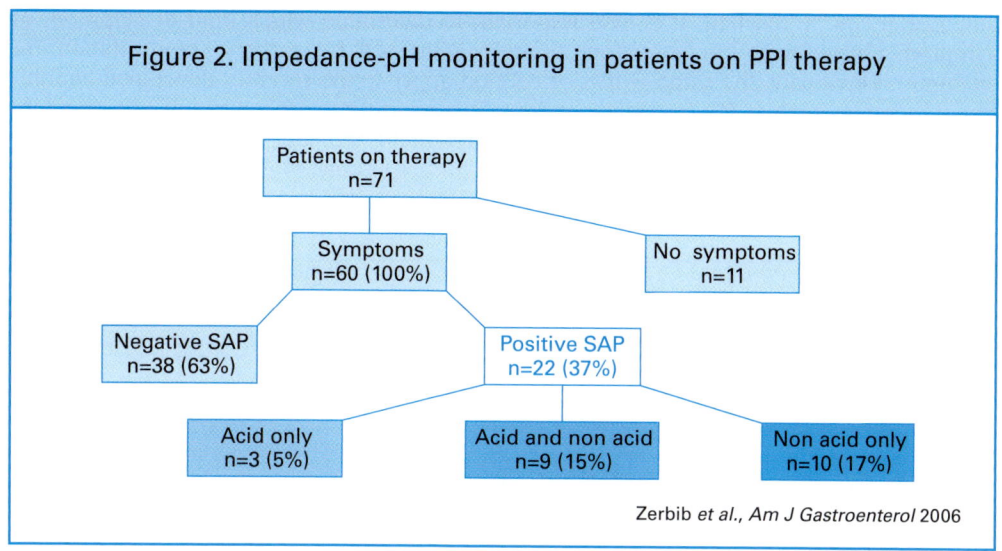

Figure 2. Impedance-pH monitoring in patients on PPI therapy

Zerbib et al., Am J Gastroenterol 2006

In other individuals, the symptoms are not acid-related; this may be the case in patients with persistent DGOR whilst on PPI therapy. One of the most attractive therapeutic approaches in these patients is to reduce the number of TLOSRs using compounds such as GABAB agonists (*e.g.* baclofen). A combination of baclofen and a PPI has been shown to be useful in some patients with refractory symptoms *(Figure 3)*. Unfortunately it is usually at the cost of significant side effects. In the future, new compounds such as specific glutamate ligands may be more adapted to this goal. Other reports using prokinetics or mucosal protectors are either anecdotal or negative. For example, tegaserod, the latest prokinetic developed, did not prove effective in a recent study. Although a case-by-case approach is always possible in these difficult to treat patients, any prolonged use of such components should be avoided.

Finally, what is the role of anti-reflux surgery in the treatment of non-acid reflux? Although anti-reflux surgery is probably the most effective therapy with respect to the various components of the reflux material, indications must be carefully discussed with each individual patient, fully informed of potential complications and outcomes of this type of surgery. Indeed, regarding laparoscopic anti-reflux surgery in general, several factors have been identified that may be associated with poorer outcome. Interestingly, these factors include normal acid exposure, lack of evidence that reflux is responsible for symptoms (low symptom index or SAP), a female gender, a short history of symptoms, a lack of mucosal breaks at index endoscopy (non-erosive disease) or a psychiatric profile. It is reasonable to extend, at least provisionally, these conclusions to the group of patients with non-acid reflux. In contrast, anti-reflux surgery may represent a reasonable option when pH-impedance or Bilitec investigations have convincingly established the link between non-acid reflux episodes and symptoms. Preliminary data in such well-selected patients seems encouraging, although a more prolonged follow-up is needed before any firm conclusion can be reached. It is also important to determine which kind of symptom or symptom cluster may be more appropriately addressed by surgery (regurgitation for example). Obviously, the same words of caution apply to the recently developed endoluminal therapies such as Rx-frequency energy delivery (Stretta procedure) or plications. In our opinion there is little, if any, room for such treatments outside the frame of prospective trials.

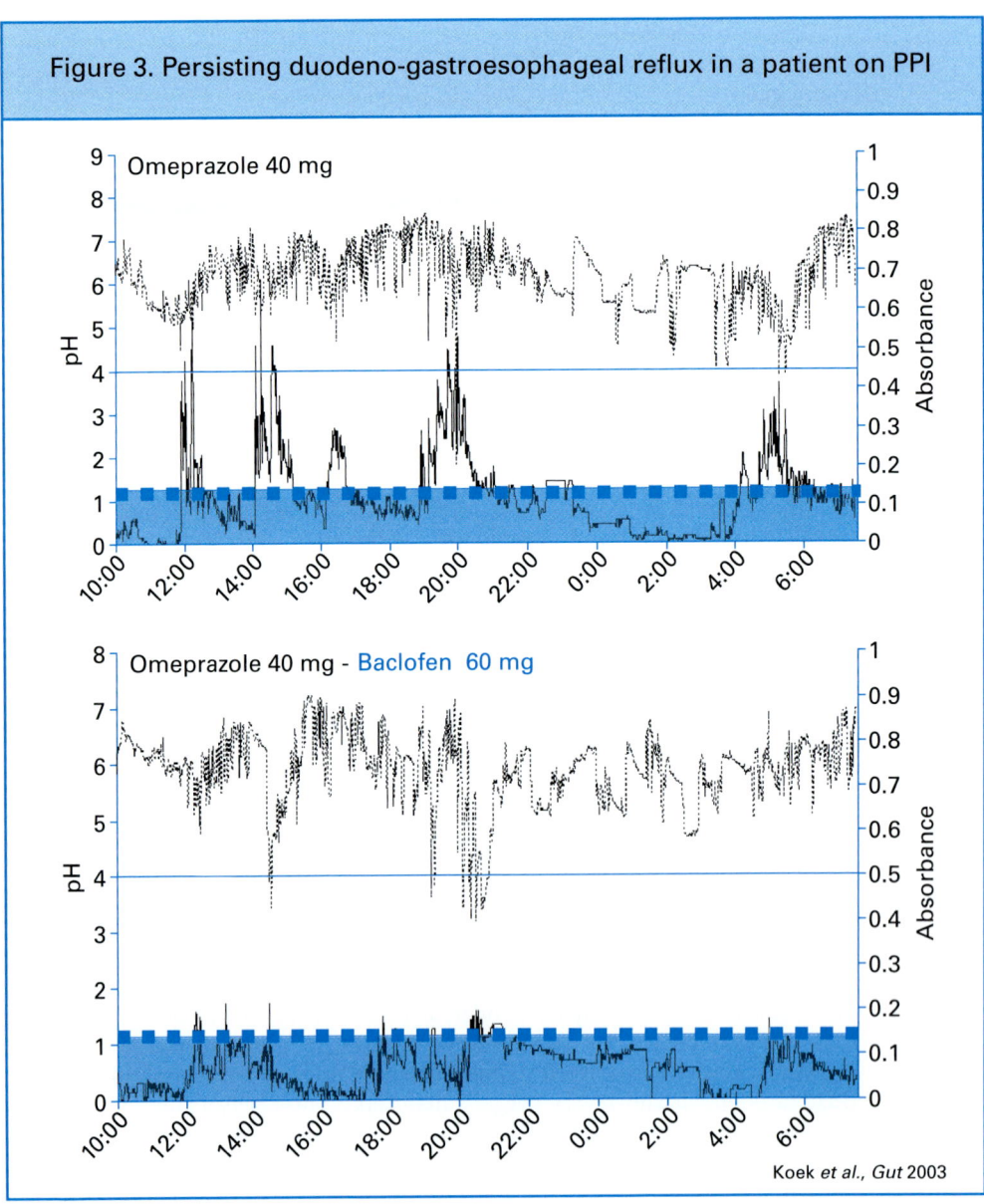

Figure 3. Persisting duodeno-gastroesophageal reflux in a patient on PPI

Koek *et al.*, *Gut* 2003

Selected references

- Champion G, Richter JE, Vaezi MF, Singh S, Alexander R. Duodenogastroesophageal reflux: relationship to pH and importance in Barrett's oesophagus. *Gastroenterology* 1994; 107: 747-54.
- Koek GH, Tack J, Sifrim D, Lerut T, Janssens J. The role of acid and duodenal gastroesophageal reflux in symptomatic GERD. *Am J Gastroenterol* 2001; 96: 2033-40.
- Koek GH, Sifrim D, Lerut T, Janssens J, Tack J. Effect of the GABAb agonist baclofen in patients with symptoms and duodeno-gastro-oesophageal reflux refractory to proton pump inhibitors. *Gut* 2003; 10: 1397-402.
- Mainie I, Tutuian R, Shay S, Vela M, Zhang X, Sifrim D, Castell DO. Acid and non-acid reflux in patients with persistent symptoms despite acid suppressive therapy: a multicenter study using combined ambulatory impedance-pH monitoring. *Gut* 2006; 55: 1398-402.
- Marshall RE, Anggiansah A, Manifold DK, Owen WA, Owen WJ. Effect of omeprazole 20 mg twice daily on duodenogastric and gastro-oesophageal bile reflux in Barrett's oesophagus. *Gut* 1998; 43: 603-6.
- Menges M, Muller M, Zeitz M. Increased acid and bile reflux in Barrett's esophagus compared to reflux esophagitis, and effect of proton pump inhibitor therapy. *Am J Gastroenterol* 2001; 96: 331-7.
- Stein HJ, Kauer WK, Feussner H, Siewert JR. Bile reflux in benign and malignant Barrett's oesophagus: effect of medical acid suppression and Nissen fundoplication. *J Gastrointest Surg* 1998; 2:333-41.
- Tack J, Koek G, Demedts I, Sifrim D, Janssens J. Gastroesophageal reflux disease poorly responsive to single-dose proton pump inhibitors in patients without Barrett's esophagus: acid reflux, bile reflux or both? *Am J Gastroenterol* 2004; 99(6): 981-8.
- Thibault R, Coron E, Sébille V, Sacher-Huvelin S, Bruley des Varannes S, Gournay J, Galmiche JP. Anti-reflux surgery for non-erosive and erosive reflux disease in community practice. *Aliment Pharmacol Ther* 2006; 24: 621-32.
- Zerbib F, Roman S, Ropert A, Bruley des Varannes S, Pouderoux P, Chaput U, Mion F, Vérin E, Galmiche JP, Sifrim D. Esophageal pH-impedance monitoring and symptom analysis in GERD: A study in patients off and on therapy. *Am J Gastroenterol* 2006; 101: 1956-63.

Irritable bowel syndrome

G. Boeckxstaens

The irritable bowel syndrome (IBS) is a prevalent functional bowel disorder characterized by abdominal pain and/or discomfort in combination with changes in bowel habits [1]. Recently, definitions have been revised and published as the Rome III criteria. In the last decade, it has become increasingly clear that patients with IBS, irrespective of the predominant bowel habit, have an increased perception of bowel distention. This so-called visceral hypersensitivity has been demonstrated in 60-95% of patients [2], and thus represents the major pathophysiological mechanism identified so far. Several hypotheses have been forwarded to explain this altered visceroperception [3, 4].

Obviously, changes in pain perception can result at any level between perception of visceral stimuli in the periphery and interpretation of afferent information in the brain. Recently, inflammation has gained a lot of attention as underlying mechanism of hypersensitivity. Especially the identification of persistent microscopic inflammation in patients with postinfectious IBS has contributed enormously to this new insight [5, 6].

By now, several different groups have confirmed the presence of microscopic mucosal inflammation in IBS [4, 7]. In addition to microscopic inflammation, increased mast cells have been demonstrated in the mucosa of IBS patients as well. Interestingly, the intensity of abdominal complaints seem to correlate with the distance between mast cells and nerve fibers [8]. Furthermore, biopsies taken from IBS patients release more tryptase and histamine, whereas the supernatant from IBS biopsies induces visceral hypersensitivity when instilled intrarectally in rodents.

The exact trigger for this increase in inflammatory cells or mast cells remains however unknown. Changes in intestinal permeability, either following infection or due to stress, may be a possible mechanism [9-11]. Increased influx of intraluminal antigens, f.e. bacterial antigens, may subsequently trigger the immune system resulting in subtle inflammation. In animal models, it is well established that inflammation changes the gain of nociceptors such as TRPV1, but clearly several other nociceptors on afferent nerve fibers may play an important role in visceral hypersensitivity. Other possible mechanisms leading to abnormal pain perception may be upregulation of spinal neurons, or abnormal processing of afferent information in the brain [12]. Recent brain imaging studies indeed revealed activation of different brain areas in response to bowel distention in IBS patients compared to healthy controls. Further studies identifying the underlying mechanisms and the receptors/mediators involved are of crucial importance for the development of more efficient drugs.

Selected references

1. Talley NJ, Zinsmeister AR, Melton LJ, III. Irritable bowel syndrome in a community: symptom subgroups, risk factors, and health care utilization. *Am J Epidemiol* 1995; 142: 76-83.
2. Mertz H, Naliboff B, Munakata J, Niazi N, Mayer EA. Altered rectal perception is a biological marker of patients with irritable bowel syndrome. *Gastroenterology* 1995; 109: 40-52.
3. Mayer EA. Emerging disease model for functional gastrointestinal disorders. *Am J Med* 1999; 107: 12S-19S.
4. Spiller RC. Inflammation as a basis for functional GI disorders. *Best Pract Res Clin Gastroenterol* 2004; 18: 641-61.
5. Spiller RC. Postinfectious irritable bowel syndrome. *Gastroenterology* 2003; 124: 1662-71.
6. Spiller RC, Jenkins D, Thornley JP, Hebden JM, Wright T, Skinner M, Neal KR. Increased rectal mucosal enteroendocrine cells, T lymphocytes, and increased gut permeability following acute Campylobacter enteritis and in post-dysenteric irritable bowel syndrome. *Gut* 2000; 47: 804-11.
7. Barbara G, De GR, Stanghellini V, Cremon C, Corinaldesi R. A role for inflammation in irritable bowel syndrome? *Gut* 2002; 51 (Suppl. 1): i41-i44.
8. Barbara G, Stanghellini V, De GR, Cremon C, Cottrell GS, Santini D, Pasquinelli G, Morselli-Labate AM, Grady EF, Bunnett NW, Collins SM, Corinaldesi R. Activated mast cells in proximity to colonic nerves correlate with abdominal pain in irritable bowel syndrome. *Gastroenterology* 2004; 126: 693-702.
9. Barbara G. Mucosal barrier defects in irritable bowel syndrome. Who left the door open? *Am J Gastroenterol* 2006; 101: 1295-8.
10. Ferrier L, Berard F, Debrauwer L, Chabo C, Langella P, Bueno L, Fioramonti J. Impairment of the intestinal barrier by ethanol involves enteric microflora and mast cell activation in rodents. *Am J Pathol* 2006; 168: 1148-54.
11. Barreau F, Ferrier L, Fioramonti J, Bueno L. Neonatal maternal deprivation triggers long term alterations in colonic epithelial barrier and mucosal immunity in rats. *Gut* 2004; 53: 501-6.
12. Mayer EA, Collins SM. Evolving pathophysiologic models of functional gastrointestinal disorders. *Gastroenterology* 2002; 122: 2032-48.

Systematic review of sacral nerve stimulation for faecal incontinence and constipation*

Michael A. Kamm et al.

St Mark's Hospital, Harrow, UK

Background and method

This systematic review assesses the efficacy and safety of sacral nerve stimulation (SNS) for faecal incontinence and constipation. Electronic databases and selected websites were searched for studies evaluating SNS in the treatment of faecal incontinence or constipation. Primary outcome measures included episodes of faecal incontinence per week (faecal incontinence studies) and number of evacuations per week (constipation studies).

Results

From 106 potentially relevant reports, six patient series and one crossover study of SNS for faecal incontinence, and four patient series and one crossover study of SNS for constipation, were included. After implantation, 41-75 per cent of patients achieved complete faecal continence and 75-100 per cent experienced improvement in episodes of incontinence. There were 19 adverse events among 149 patients. The small crossover study reported increased episodes of faecal incontinence when the implanted pulse generator was switched off. Case series of SNS for constipation reported an increased frequency of evacuation. There were four adverse events among the 20 patients with a permanent implant. The small crossover study reported a reduced number of evacuations when the pulse generator was switched off.

---

* Reproduced with permission from *Br J Surg* 2004 ; 91 : 1559-69.

Conclusion

SNS results in significant improvement in faecal incontinence in patients resistant to conservative treatment. Early data also suggest benefit in the treatment of constipation.

Selected references

- Ferulano GP, La Manna S, Dilillo S. Sacral neuromodulation in fecal continence disorders. *Recenti Prog Med* 2002; 93: 403-9.
- Leroi AM. Neuromodulation of the sacral roots and fecal incontinence. *Hepatogastroenterology* 2000; 7: 453-8.
- Matzel KE. Sacral spinal nerve stimulation. *Chirurg* 2001; 17: 230-6.
- Matzel KE, Stadelmaier U, Gall FP. Direct electrostimulation of sacral spinal nerves within the scope of the diagnosis of anorectal function. *Langenbecks Arch Chir* 1995; 380: 184-8.
- Matzel KE, Stadelmaier U, Hohenfellner M, Gall FP. Permanent electrostimulation of sacral spinal nerves with an implantable neurostimulator in treatment of fecal incontinence. *Chirurg* 1995; 66: 813-7.
- Matzel KE, Stadelmaier U, Hohenfellner M, Hohenberger W. Treatment of insufficiency of the anal sphincter by sacral spinal nerve stimulation with implantable neurostimulators. *Langenbecks Arch Chir Suppl Kongressbd* 1998; 115: 494-7.
- Michot F, Leroi AM. Sacral nerve stimulation: promising treatment for anal incontinence? *Ann Chir* 2002; 127: 247-9.
- National Institute for Clinical Excellence. Sacral nerve stimulation for faecal incontinence. IP Guidance Number IPG 0005. http://www.nice.org.uk/cms/ip/ipcat.aspx? c = 56890 [May 2003].
- Rasmussen OO, Christiansen J. Sacral nerve stimulation in fecal incontinence. *Ugeskr Laeger* 2002; 164: 3866-8.
- Sielezneff I, Pirro N, Ouaissi M, Cesari J, Consentino B, Sastre B. Surgical treatment of anal incontinence. *Ann Chir* 2002; 127: 670-9.
- Uludag O, Darby M, Dejong CH, Shouten WR, Baeten CG. Sacral neuromodulation is effective in the treatment of fecal incontinence with intact sphincter muscles; a prospective study. *Ned Tijdschr Geneeskd* 2002; 146: 989-93.

Conventional *versus* robot-assisted thoraco(laparo)scopic esophagolymphadenectomy for esophageal cancer

Judith Boone, Inne H.M. Borel Rinkes, Richard van Hillegersberg

Department of Surgery, University Medical Center Utrecht, The Netherlands

The incidence of esophageal cancer in the Western world is rapidly increasing, mainly due to a rise in adenocarcinoma [1]. Surgical tumor resection with lymph node dissection offers the only chance for cure, with an overall 5-year survival rate of 20%.

Open transthoracic and transhiatal esophagolymphadenectomy

A randomized Dutch multicentric study has compared the 2 open surgical approaches and has shown a strong trend towards a survival benefit for the transthoracic approach comprising extended lymph node dissection, compared to the limited transhiatal approach. The 5-year survival rate was 39% *versus* 29% respectively [2]. Nevertheless, this gain in survival was at the cost of a significant perioperative morbidity. Pulmonary complications occurred in 57% after transthoracic esophagectomy and in 27% after transhiatal resection. Medium stay at the intensive care unit was 6 *versus* 2 days.

To improve outcome of esophagolymphadenectomy, the oncologic outcome of a transthoracic approach should be combined with the limited morbidity of a transhiatal approach. This could be achieved by performing minimally invasive thoracoscopic esophagolymphadenectomy.

Minimally invasive surgical approaches

The world's largest series of thoracolaparoscopic esophagectomy, performed by the group of Luketich from Pittsburgh, has shown major improvements in peri-operative morbidity and mortality rates [3]. Pulmonary complication rate was 22%, compared to 57% after the open transthoracic approach. In-hospital mortality was 1.7% compared to 4%.

However, overall survival of these patients was comparable to the open limited transhiatal approach. This could be explained by the fact that an extended tumor resection or mediastinal lymph node dissection cannot be performed with conventional scopic techniques. Technical restrictions, such as 2-dimensional vision and a decrease in degrees of freedom of motion limit the extended mediastinal lymph node disection.

Robot-assisted thoracoscopic esophagolymphadenectomy

Robotic systems have been developed to overcome the limitations of conventional scopic surgery. Advantages of robotic systems are a 3-dimensional view, restoration of the natural eye-hand axis and an increased dexterity due to articulated instruments.

In specialized centers, the robot is used to support delicate scopic surgical procedures. Robotic systems may also be of added value in thoracoscopic esophageal cancer surgery, for example the dissection along vital structures as the aorta or the pulmonary vein.

During the presentation, a video will be shown to clarify the surgical procedure. In short, the entire thoracic esophagus from diaphragm up to the thoracic inlet is mobilised by robot-assisted thoracoscopy [4]. Surrounding mediastinal lymph nodes are dissected en bloc with the esophagus. After the thoracoscopic phase, *via* laparotomy or laparoscopy, the stomach is mobilized, a gastric conduit is formed and an abdominal lymph node dissection is performed. *Via* a right-sided neck incision, the neo-esophagus is anastomized to the cervical esophagus.

Results

Until January 2006, 30 patients with resectable esophageal cancer underwent robot-assisted thoracoscopic esophagolymphadenectomy using the da Vinci™ robotic system [5]. Prospectively, data was collected on patient characteristics, surgical outcome, postoperative course and histopathologic examination.

27 (90%) procedures were completed thoracoscopically. Conversion to thoracotomy occurred in 3 patients due to either extensive pulmonary adhesions, a bulky adhesive tumor in the upper esophagus, or bleeding from an aortic branch. Median operating time for the thoracoscopic phase was 180 (120-240) min and 450 (360-550) min for the complete procedure. Median blood loss was 350 (110-700) ml. after thoracoscopy and 825 (150-5300) ml at the end of surgery. A median of 20 (7-45) lymph nodes were retrieved. Median ICU stay was 4 (1-129) and postoperative ventilation time was 1 (0-126) days. Overall median hospital stay was 18 (10-182) days. Pulmonary complications occurred in 13 (43%), cardiac in 5 (17%), anastomotic leakage in 5 (17%), chylous leakage in 3 (10%) and vocal cord paralysis in 4 (13%). One (3.5%) patient died from a tracheo-neo-esophageal fistula and one from a myocardial infarction (3.5%). Pulmonary complication rate decreased markedly in the last 15 patients compared to the first 15 (33% respectively 53%) due to optimising intra-operative anaesthesiological techniques. The surgical team has experienced explicit support by the robotic system during mediastinal dissection.

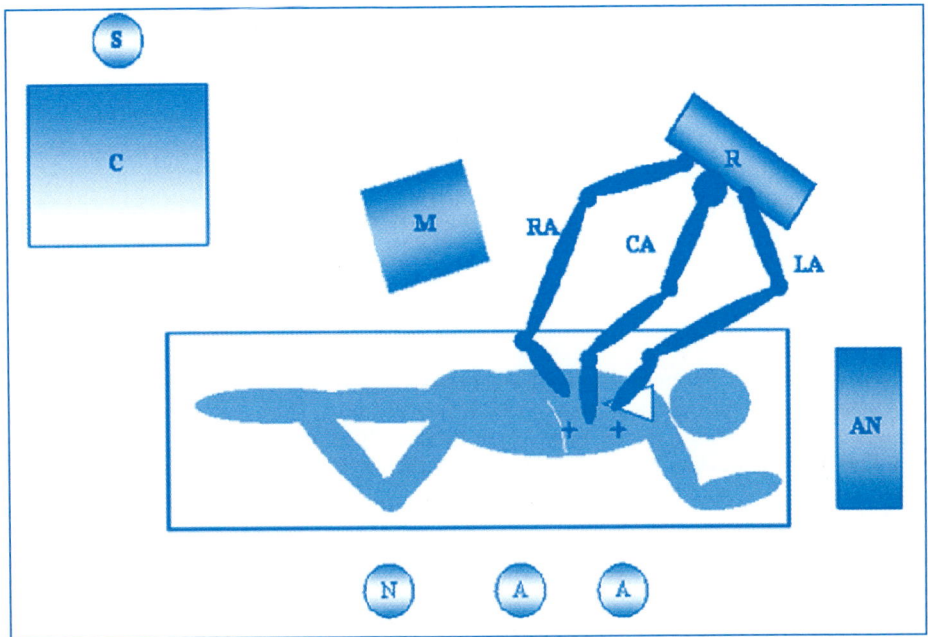

Figure 1. Set-up of the robotic system during robot-assisted thoracoscopic esophagolymphadenectomy. Adapted from [4].

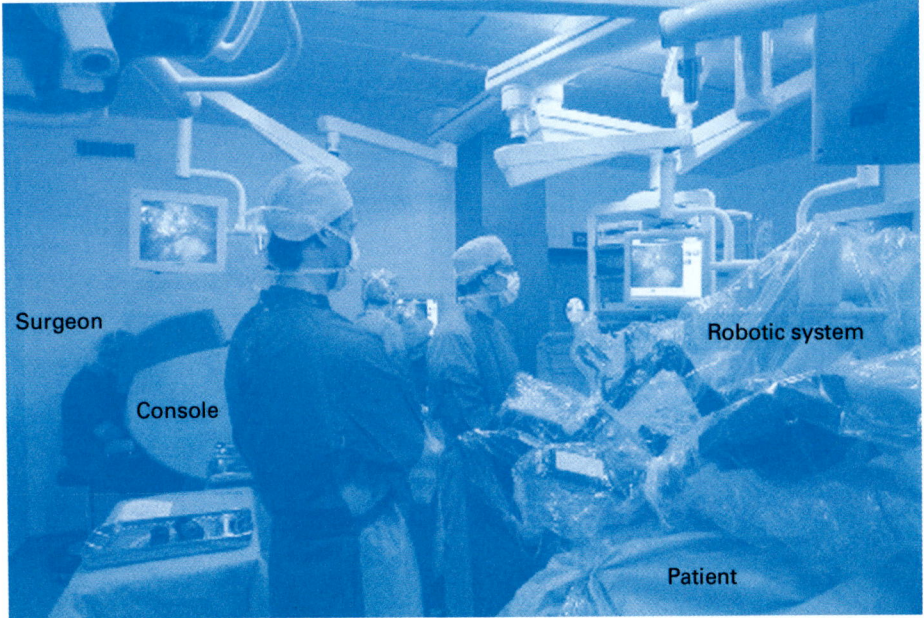

Figure 2. Positioning on the operating room. The surgeon controls the robotic system from behind the console.

Conclusion

Robot-assisted thoracoscopic esophagolymphadenectomy for cancer of the esophagus has demonstrated to be technically feasible and safe. It allows an effective mediastinal lymphadenectomy with low blood loss. Standardization of the surgical technique and increased experience should further reduce complication rate, which is at this moment in the range of the open transthoracic dissection.

References

1. Devesa SS, Blot WJ, Fraumeni JF, Jr. Changing patterns in the incidence of esophageal and gastric carcinoma in the United States. *Cancer* 1998; 83: 2049-53.
2. Hulscher JB, van Sandick JW, de Boer AG, Wijnhoven BP, Tijssen JG, Fockens P, Stalmeier PF, ten Kate FJ, van Dekken H, Obertop H, Tilanus HW, van Lanschot JJ. Extended transthoracic resection compared with limited transhiatal resection for adenocarcinoma of the esophagus. *N Engl J Med* 2002; 347: 1662-9.
3. Luketich JD, Alvelo-Rivera M, Buenaventura PO, Christie NA, McCaughan JS, Litle VR, Schauer PR, Close JM, Fernando HC. Minimally invasive esophagectomy: outcomes in 222 patients. *Ann Surg* 2003; 238: 486-94.
4. van Hillegersberg R, Boone J, Draaisma WA, Broeders IA, Giezeman MJ, Rinkes IH. First experience with robot-assisted thoracoscopic esophagolymphadenectomy for esophageal cancer. *Surg Endosc* 2006; 20: 1435-9.
5. Boone J, Draaisma WA, Broeders IA, Giezeman MJ, Borel R, I, van Hillegersberg R. Robot-assisted thoracoscopic esophago-lymphadenectomy for esophageal cancer. *J Clin Gastroenterol* 2006; 40: S176-S177.

Evaluating new diagnostic technology: a case of the Law of the Hammer?

Patrick M.M. Bossuyt

Department of Clinical Epidemiology, Biostatistics and Bioinformatics, Academic Medical Center, University of Amsterdam, The Netherlands

In an era of evidence-based medicine, diagnostic procedures cannot and should not escape a critical examination. There are genuine concerns of inappropriate technology, inappropriate use, and inappropriate application and interpretation of medical tests.

Unlike the methods and techniques for evaluating therapeutic measures, the methodology for diagnostic tests is far less developed. The current paradigm focuses on research of diagnostic accuracy, based on comparisons of test results with those from the reference standard.

Studies of diagnostic accuracy with deficiencies in design are prone to bias, and issues of design an analysis should be clearly reported. For this purpose, the STARD statement was published in 2003 in a number of major clinical journals.

Yet diagnostic accuracy is, by itself, not sufficient for making decisions about the introduction of diagnostic procedures. We need comparative studies to point out the incremental gains in diagnostic accuracy.

Ultimately, the use of diagnostic tests should be able to improve patient outcome. We will show how and when randomized and other study designs can be used to test this hypothesis. Unlike evaluations of therapy, RCT's of tests can yield invalid estimates, and the randomized design is not always efficient.

In this presentation, we will present examples from diagnostic test evaluations performed in the Academic Medical Centre in Amsterdam. These examples will be used to demonstrate limitations and flaws in the diagnostic accuracy paradigm.

Selected references

- Bossuyt PM, Irwig L, Craig J, Glasziou P. Comparative accuracy: assessing new tests against existing diagnostic pathways. *Br Med J* 2006; 332: 1089-92.
- Bossuyt PM, Lijmer JG, Mol BW. Randomised comparisons of medical tests: sometimes invalid, not always efficient. *Lancet* 2000; 356: 1844-7.
- Bossuyt PM, Reitsma JB, Bruns DE, Gatsonis CA, Glasziou PP, Irwig LM, Lijmer JG, Moher D, Rennie D, de Vet HC. Standards for Reporting of Diagnostic Accuracy. Towards complete and accurate reporting of studies of diagnostic accuracy: The STARD Initiative. *Radiology* 2003; 226: 24-8.
- Knottnerus JA. *Evidence Base of Clinical Diagnosis.* London: BMJ Publishing Group, 2001.
- Lijmer JG, Mol BW, Heisterkamp S, Bonsel GJ, Prins MH, van der Meulen JH, Bossuyt PM. Empirical evidence of design-related bias in studies of diagnostic tests. *JAMA* 1999; 282: 1061-6.
- Pepe M. *The Statistical Evaluation of Medical Tests for Classification and Prediction.* London: Oxford Statistical Science Series, 2004.
- Sackett DL, Haynes RB. The architecture of diagnostic research. *Br Med J* 2002; 324: 539-41.
- Whiting P, Rutjes AW, Reitsma JB, Glas AS, Bossuyt PM, Kleijnen J. Sources of variation and bias in studies of diagnostic accuracy: a systematic review. *Ann Intern Med* 2004; 140: 189-202.

Positron emission tomography *versus* computed tomography in gastrointestinal malignancies

M. Westerterp, J.J.B. van Lanschot

Computed tomography (CT) has long been the mainstay of morphologic imaging in several malignancies. It has a high diagnostic accuracy in clinical TNM staging. In recent years, functional metabolic ^{18}F-Fluorodeoxyglucose positron emission tomography (FDG-PET) has emerged as a useful tool in clinical oncology [1]. Although CT generally has been considered the state-of-the-art diagnostic modality for monitoring nonsurgical therapy in solid tumours (RECIST criteria) [2], also in this field, FDG-PET is gaining ground, because metabolic abnormalities usually precede a structural change. The interpretation of PET in abdominal images is often challenging because of the biodistribution of FDG, as physiologic uptake in a variety of abdominal/pelvic organs can make it difficult to distinguish benign from malignant uptake. Stomach wall uptake for example is common, and colonic wall uptake may be intense, especially in the coecum and rectosigmoid. The liver has a mottled appearance and moderate uptake. Lymphoid tissue often demonstrates increased uptake.

Oesophageal cancer

In recent years, FDG-PET has shown to be a useful adjunct to detect occult metastatic disease in oesophageal cancer (improvement of detection of stage IV disease in 3-20% of patients) [3]. The results of a large prospective nonrandomised trial, investigating the additional value of FDG-PET in detecting distant metastases in potentially curable patients after conventional work-up (including US of the neck, EUS and multislice CT of the neck, thorax and abdomen) showed upstaging in 7% of the patients with clinical stage III-IV disease (unpublished data). Therefore it was concluded that EUS combined with multislice CT remains the mainstay of initial staging and limited use of FDG-PET should be considered in selected patients. Regarding the role of FDG-PET in the assessment of response to neoadjuvant therapy in patients with oesophageal cancer, PET seems a promising noninvasive tool [4]. Even early in the course of therapy, there is a strong relation between tumour response and decrease in FDG uptake [5].

Colorectal cancer

Surgical resection is the preferred treatment for colorectal cancer. To determine the need for neoadjuvant treatment for rectal carcinomas preoperative imaging with abdominal CT and endorectal ultrasound is the standard of care. However, the use of CT in the preoperative management of patients with cancer of the intraperitoneal colon remains controversial. CT is often used to assist in operative planning of colon cancers, but its cost-effectiveness is unclear. Also FDG-PET has no established role in the preoperative staging of colorectal cancer, because a wide range of nonmalignant conditions show increased FDG uptake, such as inflammatory bowel disease and diverticulitis. However, assessment of the overall burden FDG uptake in the primary tumour before starting chemotherapy is a useful tool to determine appropriate response to treatment on follow up scans.

Hepatic dissemination is a common event of colorectal carcinoma. Sensitivity of helical CT scan and ultrasound for colorectal metastases is less than 85% (range 66% to 84%) [6].

Early data suggest that PET scan has a high sensitivity (95%) for detecting colorectal livermetastases but this needs further evaluation. Regarding the value of CT in monitoring response to neoadjuvant therapy in patients with colorectal liver metastases, Benoist *et al.* showed in 38 patients (with 183 lesions) that complete response on CT scan did not mean complete pathological response [7]. Initial results of assessment of residual liver metastases after neoadjuvant therapy with FDG-PET seem encouraging. A small study of 18 patients showed a significant difference in FDG-uptake between responders and nonresponders.

Gastrointestinal stromal tumours (GIST)

GISTs are uncommon tumours of the gastrointestinal tract. Most GISTs are characterized by an abnormality in c-kit and the presence of PDG-FRA α(platelet derived growth factor receptor alpha). These particular characteristics have led to the treatment with imatinib mesylate (Gleevac). Contrast-enhanced CT is able to differentiate between benign an malignant lesions. Results of available literature are conflicting; some studies show similar findings in FDG-PET images and CT, while others found that better prognostic information was supplied by FDG-PET images. Because 15 per cent of GISTs do not respond to Gleevec, it is important to assess response to Gleevac treatment. Stroobants *et al.* performed a study in 21 patients (17 GIST, 4 other soft tissue sarcomas) to evaluate if FDG-PET could be used for the early evaluation of response to imatinib mesylate treatment [8]. PET response was compared to CT (RECIST) [1]. Thirteen GISTs showed PET response, while CT response was observed in 10 of these patients after a median follow up of 8 weeks. Moreover PET response was also associated with a longer progression-free survival (92% *versus* 12% at 1 year, $p = 0.001$). Therefore it was concluded that FDG-PET is an early and sensitive method to evaluate an early response to imatinib treatment.

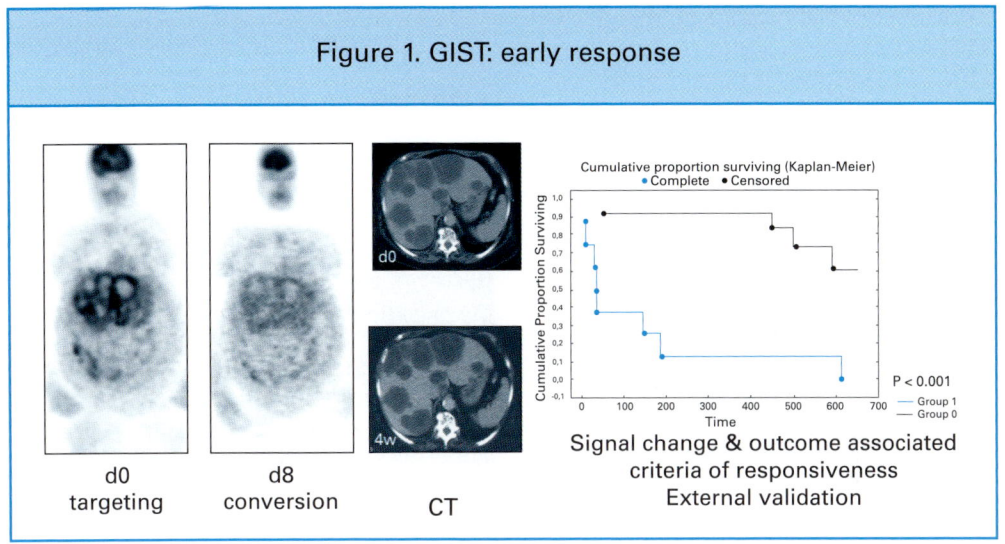

Figure 1. GIST: early response

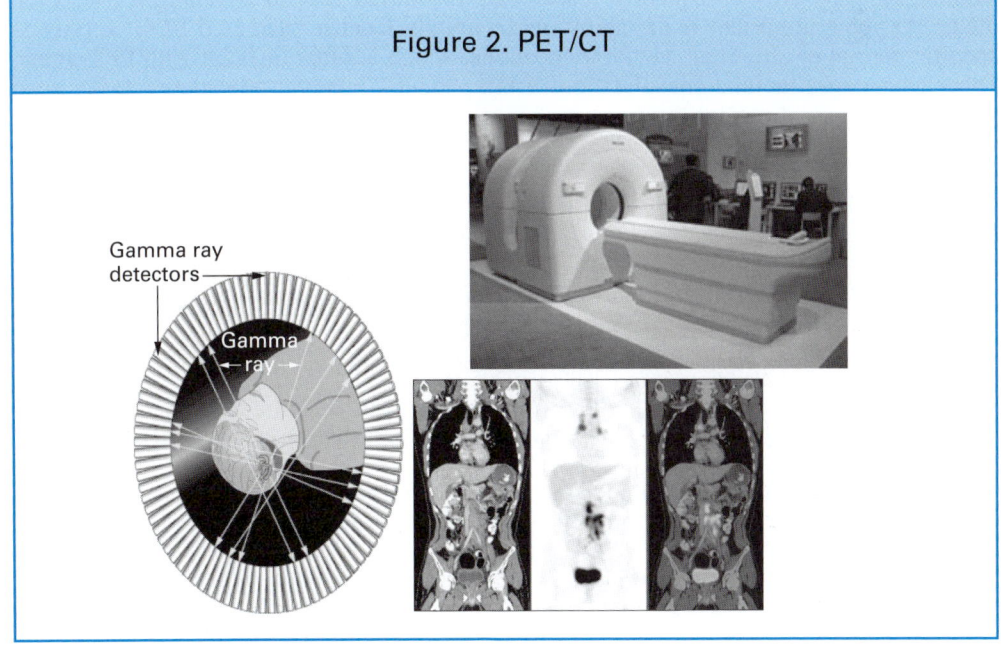

Figure 2. PET/CT

Figure 3. Indications GE

- Recurrent colorectal carcinoma
- dd recurrent disease/fibrosis
  - Increasing CEA
  - Metastases (liver, abd, lung)
  - High sens (95%) and spec (95%)
- Primary CRC: PET-CT 20% change of management

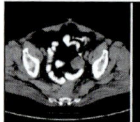
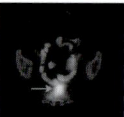
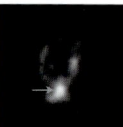
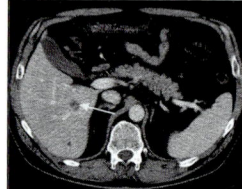
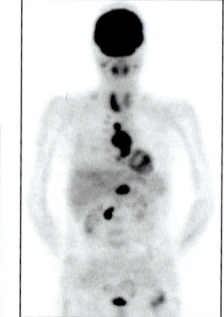

PET/CT

At this moment combined PET-computed tomography (CT), a relatively novel imaging technique, is increasingly implemented as a method for whole body oncological imaging [9]. PET/CT is a unique combination of the cross-sectional anatomic information provided by CT and the metabolic information provided by PET, which are acquired during a single examination and are subsequently fused. PET/CT offers several advantages over PET alone; the most important is the ability to accurately localise increased FDG activity at specific normal or abnormal anatomic locations, which is often difficult with PET alone. Other advantages include consolidation of the patient's imaging procedures, faster scan times and increased patient throughput.

References

1. Esteves FP, Schuster DM, Halkar RK. Gastrointestinal tract malignancies and positron emission tomography: an overview. *Semin Nucl Med* 2006; 36: 169-81.
2. Therasse P, Arbuck SG, Eisenhauer EA, *et al.* New guidelines to evaluate the response to treatment in solid tumours. *J Natl Cancer Inst* 2000; 92: 205-16.
3. van Westreenen HL, Westerterp M, Bossuyt PMM. Systematic review of the staging performance of 18F-fluorodeoxyglucose positron emission tomography in oesophageal cancer. *J Clin Oncol* 2004; 22: 3805-12.
4. Westerterp M, van Westreenen HL, Reitsma JB. Esophageal cancer: CT, endoscopic US, and FDG PET for assessment of response to neoadjuvant therapy-systematic review. *Radiology* 2005; 236: 841-51.
5. Wieder HA, Brucher BL, Zimmermann F, *et al.* Time course of tumor metabolic activity during chemoradiotherapy of esophageal squamous cell carcinoma and response to treatment. *J Clin Oncol* 2004; 22: 900-8.

6. Bipat S, van Leeuwen MS, Comans EFI, *et al.* Colorectal liver metastases: CT, MR Imaging, and PET for diagnosis, a meta-analysis. *Radiology* 2005; 237: 123-31.
7. Benoist S, Brouquet A, Penna C, *et al.* Complete response of colorectal liver metastases after chemotherapy: does it mean cure? *J Surg Oncol* 2006; 24: 3939-45.
8. Stroobants S, Goeminne J, Seegers M, *et al.* 18FDG-Positron emission tomography for the early prediction of response in advanced soft tissue sarcoma treated with imatinib mesylate (Gleevec). *Eur J Cancer* 2003; 39: 2012-20.
9. Shreve P. Establishing a PET/CT practice. *Am J Roentgenol* 2005; 184: 146-51.

Magnetic resonance cholangiopancreatography *versus* endoscopic retrograde cholangiopancreatography in HPB diseases

Myriam Delhaye

Department of Gastroenterology, Erasme Hospital, Brussels, Belgium

Endoscopic retrograde cholangiopancreatography (ERCP) was first reported in 1968, therapeutic endoscopy was first introduced in 1974 and magnetic resonance cholangiopancreatography (MRCP) has been applied since the 1990s as a potent diagnostic tool for investigation of the biliary tree and pancreatic duct system [1].

Recent studies obtained MRCP images of diagnostic quality in about 97% of cases and achieved a very high diagnostic accuracy (more than 90%) for recognition of normal biliary and pancreatic ducts, ductal dilatation and stricture, intraductal filling defects both for the bile ducts and pancreatic ducts [2].

Diagnostic information of MRCP is actually considered as equivalent to that of ERCP.

Technical features

Fluids have very long T_1 and T_2 relaxation times and appear as very low signal (= dark) on T_1-weighted images and as very high signal (= bright) on T_2-weighted images. So, heavily T_2-weighted imaging displays static fluid-filled structures with a high signal intensity and gives images similar to ERCP [3].

Exogenous secretin stimulates the secretion of fluid and bicarbonate by the exocrine pancreas and therefore improves delineation of the main pancreatic duct (MPD), Santorini duct and side branches. It increases the accuracy of MRCP in detecting pathologic stenosis of the MPD by reducing the incidence of false-positive narrowing of the MPD.

It allows a better visualization of a possible communication between the pancreatic ductal system and cystic lesions, and a better detection of anatomical variants such as pancreas divisum. Moreover, by measuring the volume of fluid in the duodenum after secretin administration it provides a specific estimation of the pancreatic exocrine function [4].

Secretin administration is safe, even in the setting of acute pancreatitis but additional time and cost are required, therefore restricting the use of secretin in warranted indications (*i.e.* assessment of early stage of chronic pancreatitis or recurrent acute pancreatitis, suspicion of pancreatic ductal disruption, differential diagnosis of pancreatic cystic tumors...).

Advantages and limitations of MRCP *(Figure 1)*

MRCP is a safe, non invasive, outpatient technique, which does not require iodinated contrast medium injection, sedation or analgesia, and without radiation exposure.

Image acquisition is possible within a few seconds, in real physiologic conditions, and with an excellent interobserver agreement. However, whereas expertise and experience may impact the accuracy of MRCP, it remains less operator dependent and less expensive than ERCP.

The main advantages of MRCP over ERCP are the complete ductal visualization above the site of ductal obstruction or disruption, the possible diagnostic information even in cases where the papilla can not be reached endoscopically (*i.e.* Billroth II gastrectomy, Roux-en-Y anastomosis, duodenal stricture or invasion, periampullary diverticulum), and the additional findings provided by the combination of non-enhanced and gadolinium-enhanced cross-sectional imaging sequences, the functional imaging, the MR angiography and the secretin-enhanced MRCP giving a complete assessment of both ductal and parenchymal diseases but also of extraductal diseases.

Figure 1. Advantages and limitations of MRCP

Advantages?	Limitations?
• Safe, non invasive	• Few contraindications
• Complete ductal visualization	• Critically ill patients
• Additional findings: all-in-one procedure	• Nature of filling defects
	• Very large fluid collections

Such a complete and accurate imaging procedure may identify patients where therapeutic intervention is needed and may guide further therapeutic strategy.

Contra-indications to MRCP were recorded in up to 5% of patients and included claustrophobia, presence of metal foreign bodies (*i.e.* cardiac pacemaker, cerebral aneurysm clip, neurostimulator), excessive body mass and lack of patient cooperation [5]. Moreover, MR imaging is difficult for critically ill patients with a lot of monitoring and therapy equipment.

Limitations of this entirely diagnostic investigation are the lack of sensitivity in detecting pancreatic calcification, in determining the nature of filling defects (sludge, blood, air, mucus, stones, proteinacceous material, debris), in depicting a minor biliary ductal narrowing due to absence of duct distension by exogenous contrast medium. Fluid collections external to the pancreatic and biliary ducts such as free peritoneal ascites and very large abdominal cystic lesions limit also the quality of the MR imaging.

Advantages and limitations of ERCP *(Figure 2)*

The major field of ERCP consists in the therapeutic options provided by this procedure and including endoscopic biliary and pancreatic sphincterotomy, stones removal, dilatation of strictures, biliary and pancreatic stenting, transpapillary and transmural drainage of fluid collections.

Additional diagnostic informations can also be obtained through ERCP such as by cholangioscopy/pancreatoscopy (allowing visual inspection of the ducts to define the extension of intraductal disease, visually-guided tissue sampling, differentiation of filling defects and stricture), by tissue and secretion analysis (*i.e.* cytology/biopsy for the diagnosis of malignancy, molecular analysis of pure pancreatic juice, bile examination) and by further development of optical coherence tomography and intraductal ultrasonography [6].

Figure 2. Advantages and limitations of ERCP

Advantages?	Limitations?
• Therapeutic options	• Operator-dependent procedure
• Additional findings: tissue sampling	• Complications
	• Radiation exposure

However, ERCP is an operator-dependent procedure requiring training, experience and great expense. Initial failure rate is reported in 3-10% of cases. Moreover, it is associated to a current complication rate around 5-7% of the cases, including pancreatitis, biliary sepsis (due to overdistension of an obstructed biliary duct by contrast medium injection), bleeding, perforation and even a mortality rate round 0.1 to 0.6% [7]. It is not recommended in children and pregnant women due to the radiation exposure.

Clinical applications of MRCP *vs* ERCP *(Figure 3)*

Figure 3. Clinical applications of MRCP *vs* ERCP

- Evaluation of
  - the biliary tree to rule out bile duct stones
  - acute / chronic pancreatitis
  - pancreatic tumors and cystic lesions
  - biliary strictures
- Miscellaneous applications
  - ductal leakage
  - anastomotic stricture
  - follow-up of chronic diseases

Evaluation of the biliary tree to rule out bile duct stones *(Figure 4)*

MRCP is actually considered as the non-invasive method of choice to prevent inappropriate exploration of the bile duct in cases where interventional endoscopic therapy is unlikely (patients with low and moderate risk of common bile duct stones before laparoscopic cholecystectomy) [3].

Evaluation of acute pancreatitis

The roles of MRCP in this clinical setting are, on the one hand, to determine the cause of a single episode or of recurrent acute pancreatitis (biliary cause, anomalous union of the pancreatic and bile ducts, congenital variants such as pancreas divisum and Santorinicele, benign or malignant tumors of the biliopancreatic junction, sphincter of Oddi dysfunction...) [8] and, on the other hand, to assess the severity and the complications of acute pancreatitis (extent of necrosis, presence and extent of fluid collections in and around the pancreas, internal content and drainability of fluid collections, MPD integrity or disruption, associated vascular complications) [9].

ERCP should be confined to patients needing therapeutic ERCP.

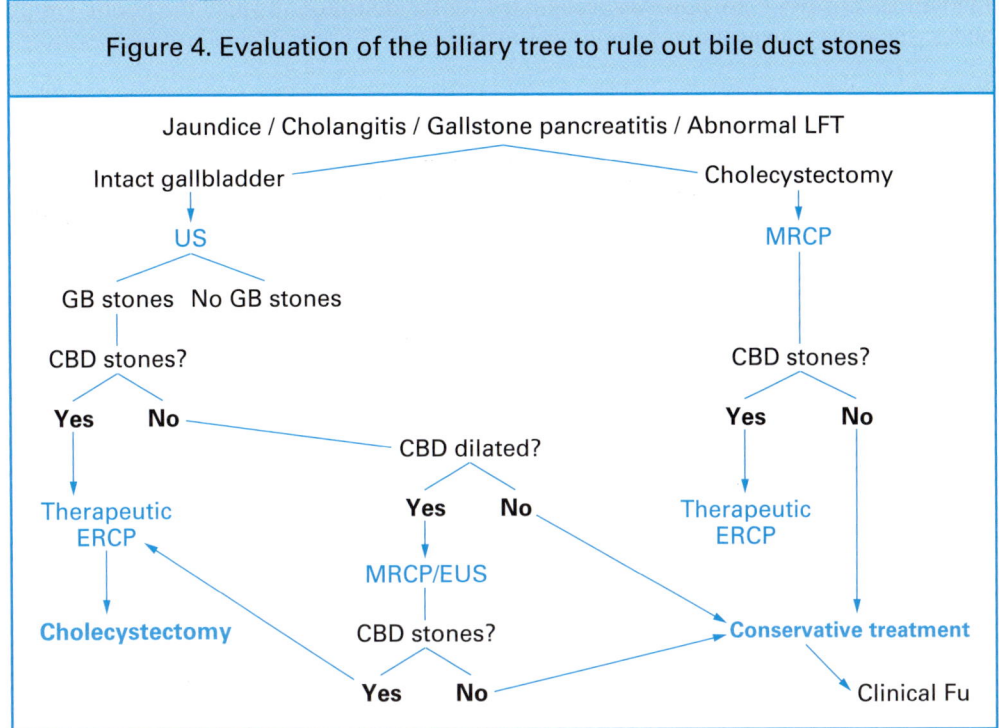

Figure 4. Evaluation of the biliary tree to rule out bile duct stones

Evaluation of chronic pancreatitis

By the combination of morphologic evaluation with functional assessment, MRCP is able to establish the diagnosis of chronic pancreatitis and to assess its complications (pseudocyst, common bile duct stricture, vascular involvement) with the aim to provide a road map before planning therapy.

Some specific features demonstrated by MRCP can suggest less frequent diagnoses such as Groove pancreatitis or autoimmune pancreatitis.

Moreover, as regards to the difficult differential diagnosis between focal inflammatory mass and pancreatic carcinoma, the study of the enhancement characteristics after gadolinium administration, the search for the "duct-penetrating sign" after secretin stimulation, and for the "double duct sign" can supply arguments in favour of malignancy [8]. On the other hand, ERCP can provide opportunity for tissue sampling and for relief of pancreatic ductal obstruction and endoscopic treatment of complications.

Evaluation of pancreatic tumors

MRCP appears as effective as ERCP for the detection of pancreatic carcinoma but has the advantage to provide, in an all-in-one imaging procedure, an accurate preoperative staging, with assessment of resectability and planning of palliative procedures or curative surgical resection [10].

Limitations of MRCP are however recognized for the detection of small metastatic lymph nodes, mesentery invasion, and peritoneal metastases.

Evaluation of pancreatic cystic lesions

Again, MRCP is a procedure of first choice to detect pancreatic cystic lesions, communicating or not with the ductal system, to assess their extension and to recognize features predictive of malignant transformation [6].

However, ERCP, by the additional information obtained from pure pancreatic juice analysis, cytological studies or biopsy from the ductal walls may define intraductal extension and confirm malignancy of specific cystic lesion like intraductal papillary mucinous tumor.

Evaluation of biliary strictures

MRCP and ERCP play complementary roles in the management of biliary strictures. Pretherapeutic MRCP is able to stratify patients according to the extent of bile duct invasion in cases of malignant hilar strictures without the risk of injecting contrast medium and may guide further endoscopic strategy.

In primary sclerosing cholangitis, dominant stricture superimposed on diffuse ductal disease may be documented by MRCP, but active ductal distension by pressure injection of contrast during ERCP may be required to reveal earlier disease [3].

Miscellaneous clinical applications of MRCP include also the detection of pancreatic or biliary ductal leakage, follow-up of chronic diseases such as primary sclerosing cholangitis, side branch type intraductal papillary mucinous tumor, follow-up of chronic pancreatitis patients after relief of ductal obstruction, detection of strictures at anastomotic sites following biliary and pancreatic surgery...

In conclusion, MRCP information provided for the diagnosis of bilio-pancreatic diseases has reduced the overall diagnostic workload of ERCP avoiding some major complications and deaths with potential cost savings [7].

ERCP should therefore be applied to patients who may benefit either from endoscopic treatment or for whom tissue sampling would be required.

References

1. ASGE guideline: the role of ERCP in diseases of the biliary tract and the pancreas. *Gastrointest Endosc* 2005; 62: 1-8.
2. Motohara T, Semelka RC, Bader TR. MR cholangiopancreatography. *Radiol Clin North Am* 2003; 41: 89-96.

3. Mac Eneaney P, Mitchell MT, Mc Dermott R. Update on magnetic resonance cholangiopancreatography. *Gastroenterol Clin North Am* 2002; 31: 731-46.
4. Matos C, Bali MA, Delhaye M, Devière J. Magnetic resonance imaging in the detection of pancreatitis and pancreatic neoplasms. *Best Practice & Research Clin Gastroenterol* 2006; 20: 157-78.
5. Ly JN, Miller FH. MR imaging of the pancreas. A practical approach. *Radiol Clin North Am* 2002; 40: 1289-306.
6. Albert JG, Riemann JF. ERCP and MRCP – when and why. *Best Practice & Research Clin Gastroenterol* 2002; 16: 399-419.
7. Farrell RJ, Noonan N, Mahmud N, Morrin MM, Kelleher D, Keeling PWN. Potential impact of magnetic resonance cholangiopancreatography on endoscopic retrograde cholangiopancreatography workload and complication rate in patients referred because of abdominal pain. *Endoscopy* 2001; 33: 668-75.
8. Fayad LM, Kowalski T, Mitchell DG. MR cholangiopancreatography: evaluation of common pancreatic diseases. *Radiol Clin North Am* 2003; 41: 97-114.
9. Arvanitakis, Delhaye M, De Maertelaere V, Bali M, Winant C, Coppens E, Jeanmart J, Zalcman M, Van Gansbeke D, Devière J, Matos C. Computed tomography and magnetic resonance imaging in the assessment of acute pancreatitis. *Gastroenterology* 2004; 126: 715-23.
10. Adamek HE, Albert JA, Breer H, Weitz M, Schilling D, Riemann JF. Pancreatic cancer detection with magnetic resonance cholangiopancreatography and endoscopic retrograde cholangiopancreatography: a prospective controlled study. *Lancet* 2000; 356: 190-3.

Achevé d'imprimer par Corlet, Imprimeur, S.A.
14110 Condé-sur-Noireau
N° d'Imprimeur : 95344 - Dépôt légal : octobre 2006
Imprimé en France